IMPROVING MEN'S HEALTH IN 30 DAYS

Support for Prostate Conditions, Erectile Dysfunction (ED), and Hormonal Imbalance in 30 Days: Rehabilitation Plan for Overall Health

By Robert Redfern

About the Author

Your Personal Health Coach
www.MyGoodHealthClub.com

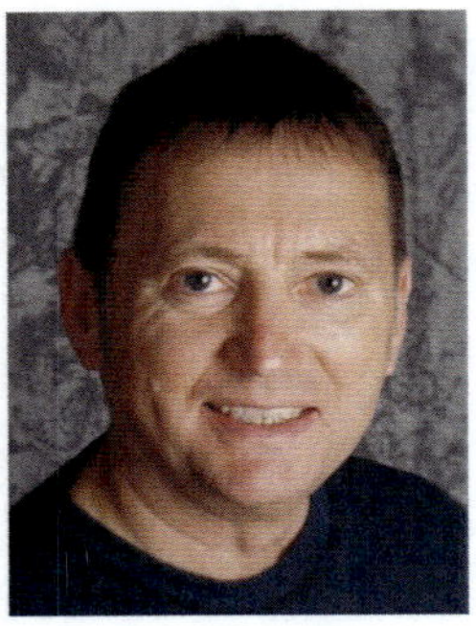

Robert Redfern was born in January 1946. He has helped thousands of people to date in more than 24 countries by providing online health guidance and resources in books, radio interviews, and TV interviews to share his nutritional discoveries. His new book series starts with *Improving Lung Health in 30 Days* and is designed to bring all of his health knowledge into one user-friendly format that anyone can understand when pursuing health recovery.

Robert became interested in health when he and his wife Anne began to take charge of their lifestyle in the late 80s. Robert had not paid much attention to his health until 1986, despite Anne's loving influence. It wasn't until Robert's parents Alfred and Marjorie died prematurely in their 60s that he was forced to re-examine his lifestyle choices.

Robert and Anne embraced a new health philosophy as they examined the health community, medical treatments, and common health issues. After researching the root cause of disease, they discovered that diet and lifestyle choices were the two most pivotal factors that contribute to overall health and well-being. Robert and Anne decided to make major changes in their diet and lifestyle, while utilizing **HealthPoint™** acupressure. The changes that they saw were exceptional.

In addition to improved health, Robert and Anne both look and feel like they have more vitality than they did decades before they started their new health plan. Currently, Robert, 69, and Anne continue to make healthy choices to live energetically and youthfully, based on a foundation of Natural Health.

ROBERT REDFERN - YOUR PERSONAL HEALTH COACH
Provides step-by-step guidance on:

Men's Health Concerns:

Prostate Conditions, Erectile Dysfunction (ED), and Hormonal Imbalance Rehabilitation in 30 Days

The Causes and the Recovery Plan

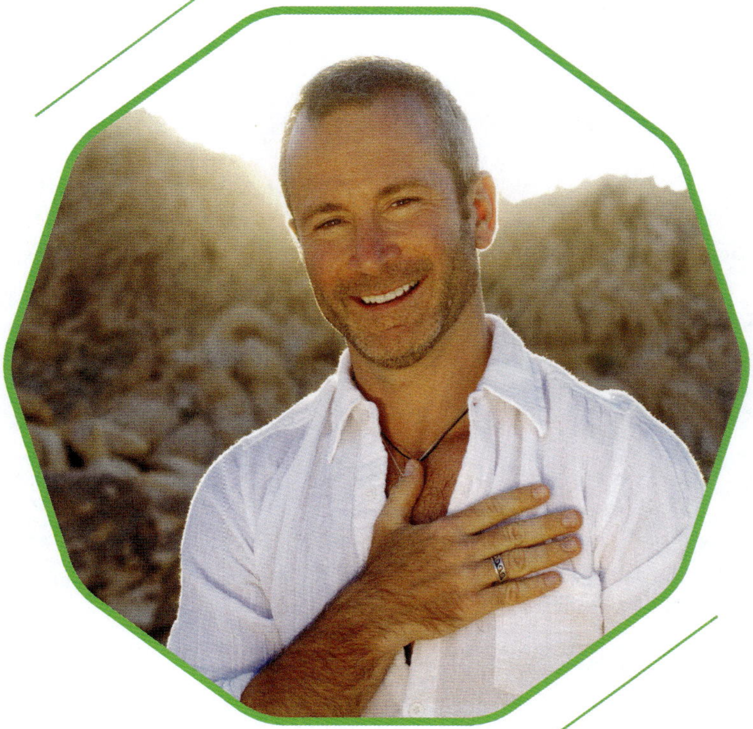

Publisher:

Naturally Healthy Publications.

Publication printed in the United Kingdom.

Publisher's Note:

This book is not intended to diagnose any disease or offer medical advice. The intention of the book is only to provide information for the reader so that they can make healthy lifestyle choices.

Warning:

Some of the information in this book may contradict advice from your physician; nonetheless, content is based on the science of natural health.

CONTENTS

Your Commitment Plan for Better Men's Health

TODAY	I DID THIS	SIGNED	DATE
I Committed	To restoring and supporting my health for all of my life.		
I Committed	To drinking 6-8 glasses of water per day with a pinch of sodium bicarbonate in each glass.		
I Committed	To spending time in the sun for 20 minutes each day (except when not advised).		
I Read	Robert's ***Improving Men's Health in 30 Days*** Book.		
I Ordered	The recommended supplements to support my plan and healing.		
I Planned	My Daily Menu using **ReallyHealthyFoods.com**		
I Started	My breathing exercises.		
I Started	Massaging the appropriate acupressure points.		
I Reread	Robert's ***Improving Men's Health in 30 Days*** Book.		
I Reviewed	The recommended supplements to support my plan and healing.		
I Reviewed	My water intake.		
I Reviewed	My Daily Menu.		
I Reviewed	My breathing exercises.		
I Reviewed	My life-giving sun exposure (except when not advised).		
I Reviewed	How to massage the appropriate acupressure points.		
I Recommitted	To restoring and supporting my health for all of my life.		
I Recommitted	To reading Robert's ***Improving Men's Health in 30 Days*** Book.		
I Recommitted	To the recommended supplements to support my plan and healing.		
I Recommitted	To my water intake.		
I Recommitted	To following my Daily Menu.		
I Recommitted	To doing my breathing exercises.		
I Recommitted	To life-giving sun exposure (except when not advised).		
I Recommitted	To massaging the appropriate acupressure points.		

Men and Their Health

Men are often taught to be strong and to keep everything inside. While this way of thinking may be beneficial in certain scenarios, it can be detrimental when it comes to health.

♂ Addressing health concerns as soon as possible is one of the keys to recovery.

Addressing the *real source* of the problem is critical. This leads us to the focus of this book: finding out what's really causing some of men's primary health concerns.

Many men are concerned about conditions that affect their sexual health. These include:

1. **Prostate health**
2. **Erectile dysfunction (ED)**
3. **Hormonal imbalances**

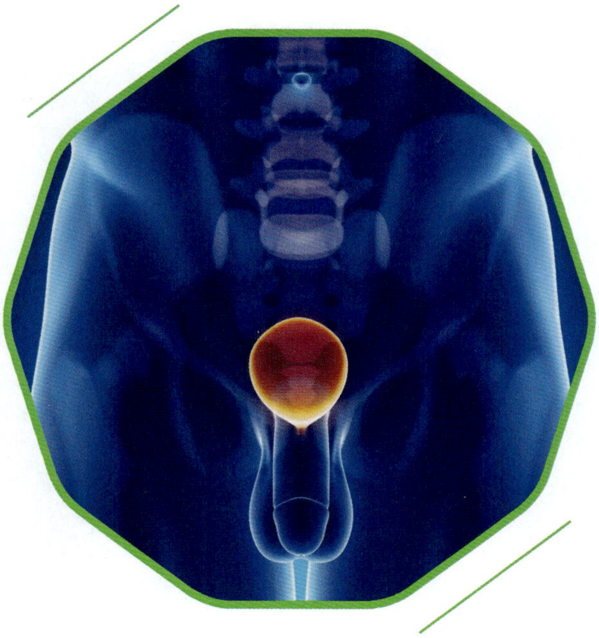

The Prostate

What Is It?

The prostate is a very small gland (about the size of a walnut), which is a component of a man's reproductive system. This gland surrounds the neck of the bladder and is responsible for secreting a portion of the fluid which makes up a man's semen.

Specifically, the prostate is located low in the pelvis, underneath the bladder, and in front of the rectum. This puts the prostate in a position where it also surrounds the urethra.

♂ "Maintaining a healthy prostate is essential to all men."

- Robert Redfern

One in three men over 40 has some kind of prostate problem. One in 13 men over 40 has a serious prostate health issue.

Prostate Conditions

There are several conditions that can affect the prostate:

1. Enlarged Prostate

The first condition is an enlarged prostate, otherwise known as Benign Prostatic Hyperplasia (BPH). An oversized prostate can create pressure on the urethra and cause problems for some men. This usually occurs after the age of 60 and can be asymptomatic for some men; however, for those who do exhibit symptoms, they may have trouble urinating and/or experience the need to urinate quite often, interfering with getting a good night's sleep.

The hormonal imbalance and chronic inflammation which lead to an enlarged prostate may be due to a number of lifestyle factors, including: infection, mineral deficiencies, not relieving oneself as soon as the sensation to urinate occurs, drinking alcoholic and caffeinated beverages, drinking any liquid within two hours before retiring for the evening, taking drugs whether prescribed or purchased at the drugstore, and consuming a diet high in unhealthy fats (saturated, hydrogenated, and trans-fats), high-sugar foods, carbohydrates, and drinks.

Treatments (Consider as a Very Last Resort)

Drugs commonly prescribed for an enlarged prostate include:

- **Alpha Blockers** - Work by giving some muscles the ability to relax—in this case, the muscles of the bladder neck and prostate. Side effects include headache, a pounding heart, nausea, weakness, and weight gain. These drugs may also change how other drugs are metabolized, increasing or decreasing their effect. When used for extended periods of time, alpha blockers may lead to a higher risk for heart failure.

- **5 Reductase Inhibitors** - Work by reducing the size of the prostate. Side effects include erectile dysfunction, decreased sex drive, abnormal ejaculation, and an increase in breast size.

Invasive surgeries for an enlarged prostate include:

- **Transurethral Resection of the Prostate (TURP) -** Surgery utilizes a resectoscope, which is put into the penis for the purpose of removing a part of the prostate.

- **Transurethral Incision of the Prostate (TUIP) -** Surgery involves going through the urethra in order to make a larger opening in the urethra and bladder.

- **Prostatectomy** - Surgery in which the lower abdomen is cut in order to enable the doctor to take out part of the prostate. The prostate may be completely removed if the doctor deems it necessary.

These prostate surgeries may lead to impotence, incontinence, blood transfusion, bleeding, infection, and urethra stricture with a recovery time of up to 8 weeks.

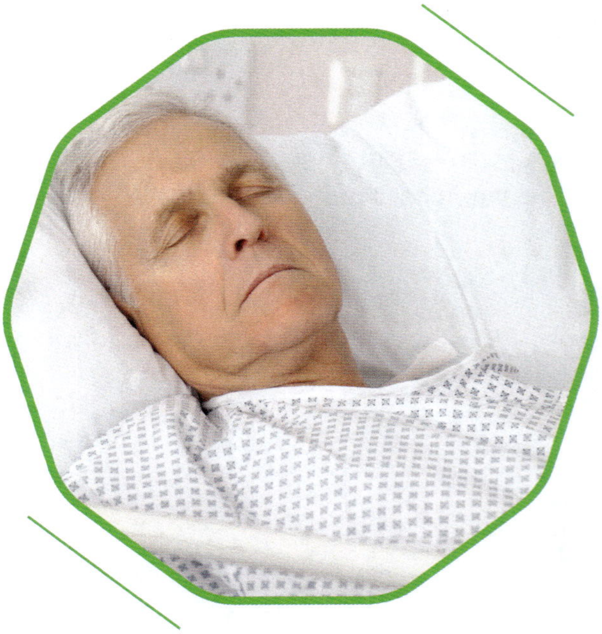

2. Prostatitis

Prostatitis is simply inflammation of the prostate. This inflammation may come with or without an infection. Prostatitis occurs in several forms: acute bacterial, chronic bacterial, and non-bacterial. Each form has some similarities, as well as some differences, in the way they are manifested. Some of the symptoms include fever, chills, lower back pain, recurring urinary tract infection, pain when urinating and ejaculating, pain in the pelvic or genital area, and a tender, swollen, inflamed prostate.

What Causes Prostatitis?

The hormonal imbalance and chronic inflammation which leads to prostatitis may be due to a number of lifestyle factors, including drinking alcoholic and caffeinated beverages, using tobacco products, eating spicy foods, drinking inadequate amounts of water, and consuming an inflammatory, high-sugar diet. It is also best to avoid sitting for long periods of time or engaging in activities which create a bounce or vibration in the body, e.g., riding a motorcycle.

Treatments (Consider as a Very Last Resort)

Drugs commonly prescribed for prostatitis include:

- **Antibiotics** - To kill infection; however, antibiotics also destroy beneficial flora in the gut, which are essential for good health.

- **Alpha Blockers** - Work by giving some muscles the ability to relax—in this case, the muscles of the bladder neck and prostate. Side effects include headache, a pounding heart, nausea, weakness, and weight gain. These drugs may also change how other drugs are metabolized, increasing or decreasing their effect. When used for extended periods of time, alpha blockers may lead to a higher risk for heart failure.

- **Pain Relievers** - In the form of non-steroidal anti-inflammatory drugs (NSAIDS), e.g., ibuprofen and aspirin. Common side effects include nausea, vomiting, diarrhea, constipation, decreased appetite, a rash, dizziness, headache, drowsiness, and gastrointestinal bleeding. NSAIDs may also damage the kidneys in those with lupus.

- **Muscle Relaxants** - Used to relax the muscles, as the name implies. Common side effects include sleepiness, a dry mouth, urinary retention, and the possibility of addiction.

A surgical option is available, depending upon the type of prostatitis. This procedure is used to open blocked ducts.

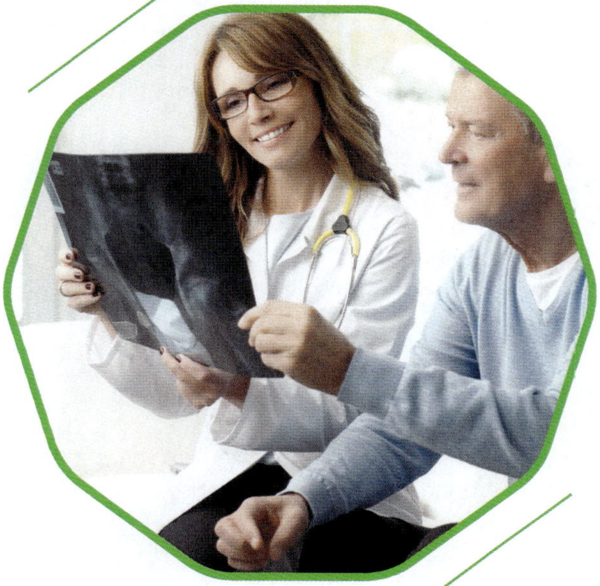

3. Prostate Cancer

Prostate cancer, like any other cancer, occurs when healthy cells begin to change (mutate) and multiply out of control, leading to a mass or tumor.

Prostate cancer deserves a little more attention here, as it is perhaps the biggest prostate concern for men. According to the World Cancer Research Fund International, prostate cancer diagnoses totaled at 1.1 million in 2012. Prostate cancer accounted for roughly 8 percent of all new cancer diagnoses and 15 percent of cancers in men.

In many Western countries, prostate cancer is one of the most common cancers and remains a leading cause of cancer death. The highest rates of prostate cancer can be found in the United States, especially among black men. China has some of the lowest rates of prostate cancer.

Signs of Prostate Cancer

Unfortunately, the vast majority of men with prostate cancer will not even notice something is wrong unless they visit their doctor and have a prostate exam, PSA screening, and/or a biopsy.

For those who do exhibit symptoms, they will notice:

- Painful urination
- Hard time voiding
- Frequent urination and retention
- Blood in the urine

3 Stages of Prostate Cancer Growth

How does prostate cancer progress and tumors grow? There are three stages of growth:

1. **Initiation** - Cancer cells are created and then destroyed as they are not needed.
2. **Promotion** - The important stage; cancer continues to grow as it is needed by the immune system, and variables needed for this growth are made available.
3. **Progression** - Quite simply, when cancer is out of control, based upon having the right conditions during the promotion stage; it is growing and spreading rapidly.

Prostate cancer can be halted and turned back by a healthy body, depending upon the causes and what changes are made to these causes.

Cancer cells are part of an interesting phenomenon. Out of the trillions of cells in our body, some of these cells are cancer cells. Yes, they are naturally present, even when we do not actually have cancer, and do not normally present a threat. A strong, healthy body and immune system will usually destroy these cancer cells, stopping them dead in their tracks before they have the chance to multiply and make us sick.

♂ A strong, healthy body and immune system are therefore crucial in preventing this dysfunction and possibly reversing cancer.

Source: Can J Urol. Feb 2008; 15(1): 3866–3871.

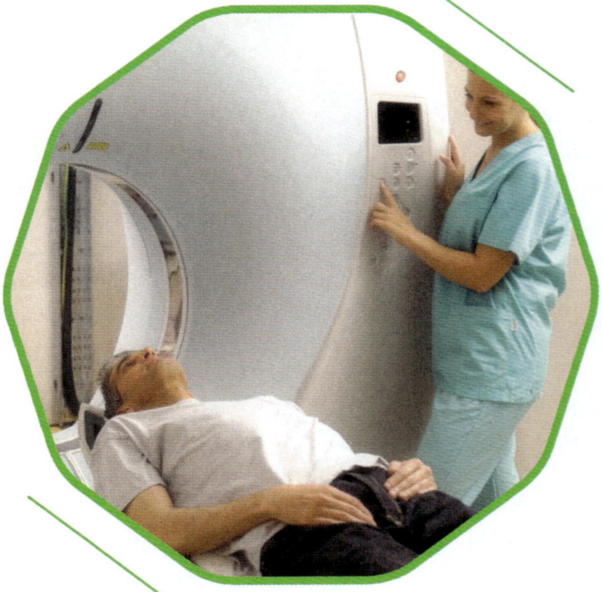

Who Gets Prostate Cancer?

Risk starts to elevate after the mid-forties, with men in their seventies showing signs of cancerous cells. While any man is a candidate, black men have the highest rates of prostate cancer, along with the highest rates of death.

Other risk factors include:

- **First degree relative (parent, child, or sibling) with prostate cancer.** Genetics may play a part in prostate cancer, though they do not have as much impact as inherited unhealthy lifestyle habits.

- **Consumption of dairy products.** Calcium from dairy foods may use up vitamin D, which has shown to be protective against prostate cancer.

- **Drinking soft drinks.** According to a study published in the *American Journal of Clinical Nutrition*, which followed 8128 men ages 45 to 73 years old over 15 years, men who drank just one 300 ml sugary soft drink a day were 40 percent more likely to develop prostate cancer.

- **Being overweight, especially obese.** Excess weight greatly increases the risk for prostate cancer, as does having another disease related to being obese, e.g., metabolic syndrome.

- **Sedentary lifestyle.** Being physically active can help control weight, and while a lack of exercise may not be an actual risk factor for prostate cancer, it seems to be a factor in the advancement of the disease.

- **Elevated IGF-1 blood levels.** IGF-1 or insulin-like growth factor-1, is a growth hormone present in animals and humans alike. Growth factors are responsible for cell growth, which can be a good thing; however, in the case of cancer cells, growth factors can perpetuate their existence and their survival.

What Causes Prostate Cancer?

Dr. Caldwell B. Esselstyn Jr., a former surgeon at the Cleveland Clinic, President of the Cleveland Clinic staff, author, and researcher, is famous for saying, "Genes load the gun, but lifestyle pulls the trigger." This is never more applicable than when it comes to prostate cancer.

While genetics do play a role in prostate cancer, what you choose to do will greatly dictate whether or not your genes will be expressed or activated. For example, all of the factors for prostate cancer, except in extremely rare cases, can be changed through the choices we make.

Even poor genes that indicate cancer can be "overwritten" by making the necessary dietary and environmental changes, according to research. Simply put, this means that your DNA is not a death sentence. Researchers from Belgrade's Institute for Medical Research assert that epigenetics trump genetics, meaning that outside influences can help to rewrite DNA coding. The very most important outside influence is diet, followed by environmental factors. Bioactive foods, particularly nutrient-rich, non-starchy vegetables, can improve health and prevent disease.

♂ So, are you doomed to have prostate cancer if it runs in your family? Certainly not!

The hormonal imbalance and chronic inflammation that lead to prostate cancer may be due to a number of lifestyle factors, including a diet high in animal products, processed foods, refined carbohydrates, oils, sodas, and excessive alcohol consumption:

- A high intake of saturated fat increased death from prostate cancer by as much as three times.

- Many prostate cancer patients actually die from cardiovascular disease before they die from cancer.

It is clear that diet plays a key role in the fight against prostate cancer. But first, it's important to understand exactly what inflammation is, and even more importantly what chronic inflammation is, as it is the foundation for most, if not all, health conditions and diseases. Addressing **chronic inflammation** is critical to the recovery of all men's health issues.

Sources:
Am J Clin Nutr December 2012 vol. 96 no. 6 1409-1418
Nutrition and Cancer, 2013; 65 (6): 781-92

What Is Inflammation?

Inflammation is a localized external or internal reaction characterized by redness, warmth, swelling, and pain due to an infection, irritation, injury, or trauma.

> ♂ *Inflammation is an entirely normal process used by the body to heal itself.*

Examples of when the body uses inflammation for healing include exposure to toxins and the presence of unwanted microorganisms. The inflammation process starts with increased blood flow to the affected area, calling in various members of the immune system. The inflammation process ends when the members of the immune system have done their job by removing and killing pathogens and healing any damaged tissue.

While inflammation is essential to life, it is also the perfect environment for infection. If not dealt with by other parts of the immune system, then cancer cells are used as a possible last resort. Cancer uses our anti-inflammatory buffer against us to promote its own protective growth.

Prostate Cancer and the Inflammation Connection

Certain cancers have a direct link to inflammation. Prior to the initiation of cancer, there is a long-term inflammatory condition setting the stage for cancer to emerge.

The process used to cause prostate cancer cell growth is the same one used to fight inflammation. Cancer cells are called out as a last resort. If the health of the body and strength of the immune system remains weak, cancer cells can become uncontrollable and with a few exceptions, e.g., leukemia, result in tumors.

> ♂ *Cancer cells become uncontrollable by the failure of the body's systems.*

What we do every day can either contribute to the proliferation of prostate cancer or help to slow down, stop, or even reverse it.

Prostate cancer usually stems from a:

- **Cancer-promoting lifestyle**
- **Compromised immune system/inflammation**

The ways to "catch" prostate cancer are one in the same. A cancer-promoting lifestyle compromises the immune system, creates inflammation, and leads to cancer.

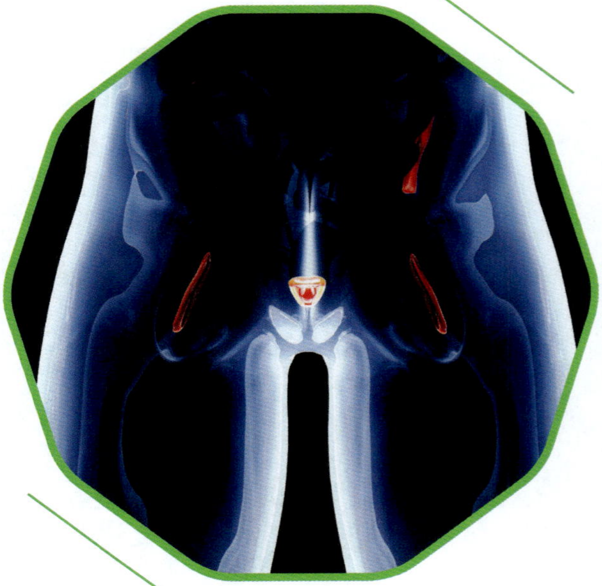

Traditional Prostate Cancer Treatments and Their Side Effects (Consider as a Very Last Resort)

As we have learned, a strong immune system is a necessary component in fighting and surviving cancer. So, what approach does the traditional treatment of cancer take?

In its steps to destroy prostate cancer, it also destroys and devastates the immune system!

Cancer treatment can be approached utilizing only one therapy or a combination. When a combination of modalities is used, these therapies can be given concurrently, consecutively, or in cycles.

The three primary prostate cancer treatments are:

1. Surgery

The purpose of surgery is to remove a tumor or tumors without compromising any bodily functions. If this is not possible, a tumor may be debulked or, in other words, removed in part. This form of surgery comes with its own set of problems. While partial removal of a tumor may increase the time a patient has to live without "curing" the cancer, it may also come with side effects—decreasing the comfort level of the patient and thus reducing their quality of life for the time they have left.

2. Chemotherapy

Chemotherapy is a systemic (affects the entire body) approach to cancer treatment. This approach generally involves administering a combination of several drugs, either through the vein or orally. While chemotherapy does kill cancer cells, it can't differentiate between killing abnormal cells and healthy cells! Healthy cells include the blood-forming stem cells found in bone marrow, which are responsible for producing components of the immune system. This often creates a need for a bone marrow transplant after treatment is completed.

Side effects of chemotherapy may include nausea and vomiting, a change in blood counts, infertility and impotence, skin irritation, hair loss, inability to clot blood, weight loss, nerve damage, fatigue, myopathy, and more.

3. Radiation

The administration of radiation therapy is done through x-ray machines, which produce substantially more energy (up to a thousand times greater) than an everyday x-ray machine. This is strong enough to wipe out cancer cells, as well as healthy cells, in the body. The use of this machine, called a linear accelerator, is localized. Tumor shrinkage is slow and may not even be apparent until well after the cessation of treatment.

Radiation side effects may include fatigue, hair loss, impotence, dry mouth, intestinal inflammation, cystitis, dermatitis, and more.

The treatment for cancer can be just as toxic as the disease itself.

An important consideration in fighting cancer is to address the source of the problem. There are cancer cells which cannot be eradicated with treatment and can therefore be reactivated when the origin of the cancer (a poor diet) is engaged in once again.

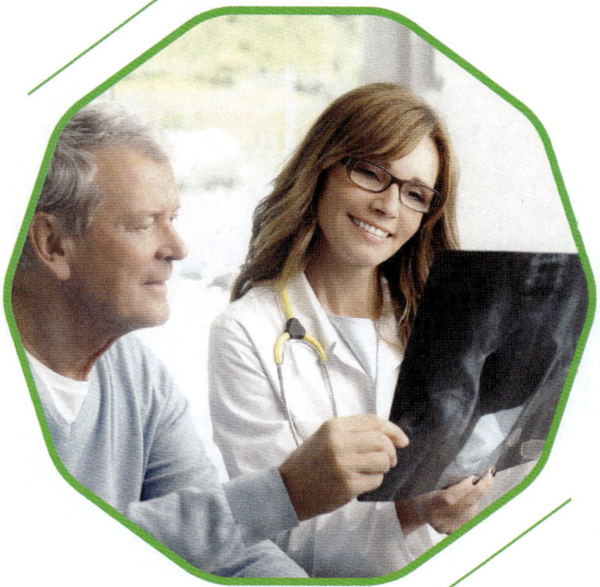

Prostate Cancer's "Miracle" Spice

Curcumin is a phytochemical and belongs to a class of compounds known as curcuminoids. Other than being an important component of turmeric, a favorite Indian spice, curcumin is a natural polyphenol, a group of chemicals which provide many health benefits. Curcumin is a standardized extract from the dried root of the curcuma plant, the root being the portion used for medicinal purposes.

The history of curcumin tells about its many uses, including its role in healing and food preparation. Curcumin, in the form of turmeric, was used as a folk remedy, as well as a cure, in ancient ayurvedic medicine. It was considered a symbol of prosperity. Curcumin was used in Indian and traditional Chinese medicine as a primary anti-inflammatory spice and as a relief for stomach irritation, dating as far back as 600 A.D.

Research now proves why ancient medicine has used curcumin for thousands of years. Even though **curcumin's chemical makeup** was determined in 1910, it took until the mid-1970s and 80s to study curcumin on a large scale.

Curcumin possesses several anti-cancer benefits that make it useful for prostate cancer prevention. One of its most recognized features is its antioxidant action. Turmeric, which contains curcumin, has traditionally been used as a food preservative for good reason: It keeps food from going rancid or oxidizing. And just as turmeric keeps oxygen from turning meat rancid, it protects our own bodies from damaging free radicals.

> ♂ *Turmeric is not curcumin - curcumin is thousands of times more powerful than simple turmeric.*

Free radicals promote cancer by damaging DNA and activating genes. Radiation damages DNA partially through free radicals. In a recent study, it was demonstrated that under laboratory conditions, curcumin could protect bacteria from a lethal dose of radiation almost perfectly. Bacterial DNA emerged virtually intact.

Curcumin may prove promising for prostate cancer. Curcumin can slow prostate cancer growth and can help protect against both prostate and breast cancers. Animal studies have confirmed that the polyphenol helps to slow tumor growth associated with prostate cancer. Researchers agree that while curcumin may not replace conventional cancer treatment, it should be part of a nutritional therapy program for anyone at risk for or suffering from breast or prostate cancer.

Source: Carcinogenesis, 2012; 33: 2507-19.

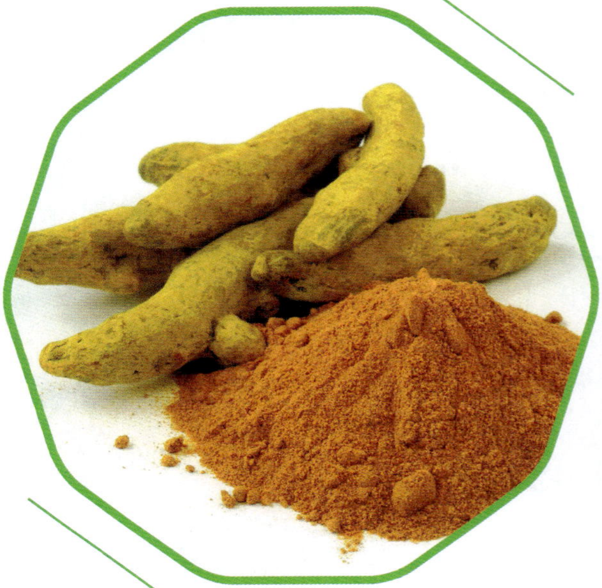

Cutting-Edge Prostate Research

Bee Pollen

Your body needs low levels of the hormone DHT to maintain a healthy-sized prostate. Unfortunately, time is not on your side.

> ♂ *DHT hormone levels increase in men with age.*

However, studies have shown that bee pollen can help to lower rising DHT levels (like pollen extract Graminex G63). When researchers in England gave bee pollen to men who used the bathroom too often or had difficulty urinating, results were noticeable. Within just six months, 79 percent of the men saw a significant improvement, and 36 percent of men were satisfied with their results. This study supports bee pollen to relax the smooth muscles in the urinary tract so that urine can flow freely once again.

Source: Rugendorff, E.W., W. Weidner, L. Ebling, and A.C. Buck. "Results of Treatment with Pollen Extract (Cernilton) in Chronic Prostatitis and Prostatodynia." British Journal of Urology. 1993.71

Grape Seed Extract

Grape seed extract is a renowned cancer-fighter. Through extensive laboratory testing, researchers have confirmed that grape seed extract can kill prostate cancer cells, while leaving healthy cells intact.

> ♂ *Grape seed's power comes from a cancer-fighting compound called B2G2.*

University of Colorado Cancer Center researchers have investigated grape seed's potency for more than 10 years. Just recently, researchers were able to isolate and identify B2G2. Further research and funding are needed to create a compound and receive FDA approval before clinical trials can begin.

Source: Nutrition and Cancer, 2013; 131105125434005

Red Meat

> ♂ *Most of us like to enjoy a nice, juicy steak after a long day of work, but your favorite meal may put your prostate health at risk.*

Research published in the journal *Carcinogenesis* confirmed that cooking red meat at high temperatures, especially when pan-fried, could increase the risk of advanced prostate cancer by up to 40 percent.

Researchers assessed data from close to 2000 men who participated in the California Collaborative Prostate Cancer Study. Based on a questionnaire completed by each participant that evaluated the amount and type of meat eaten, as well as cooking method, prostate cancer risk was determined. Throughout the course of the study, over 1000 men were diagnosed with advanced prostate cancer. Dr. Mariana Stern, lead study author, stated that men who ate more than 2.5 servings of pan-fried red meat a week cooked at high temperatures had a 40 percent greater advanced prostate cancer risk.

Source: Carcinogenesis. 2012 Nov;33(11):2108-18. doi: 10.1093/carcin/bgs242.

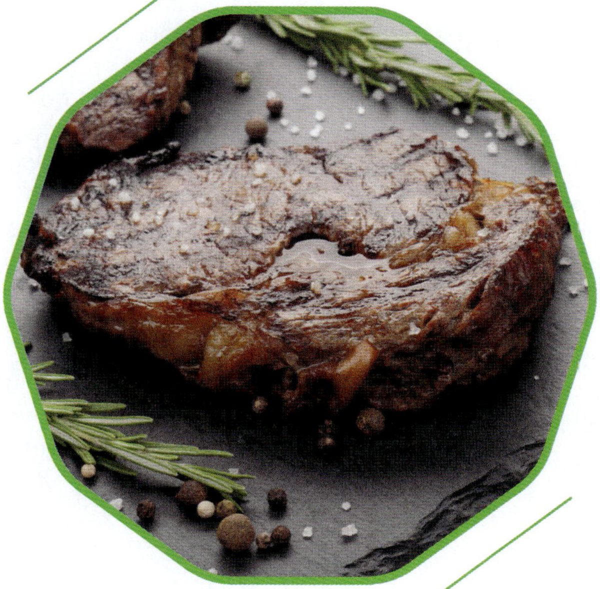

Erectile Dysfunction (ED)

Erectile dysfunction (ED), affectionately known as impotence, is a man's inability to acquire and keep an erection which is satisfactory for sexual intimacy. Ten percent of men will experience some level of ED at least once over their lifetime, with many experiencing long-term problems.

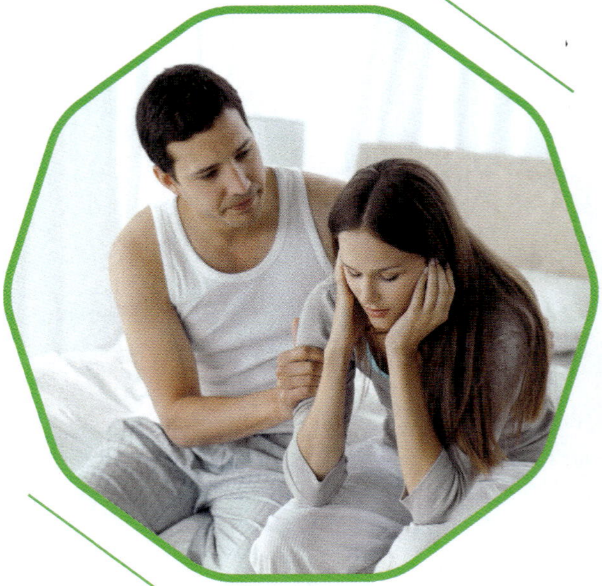

♂ How do you know if you have erectile dysfunction?

An occasional struggle with achieving an erection can be attributable to an array of issues, including stress, self-doubt, fatigue, overconsumption of alcohol, or problems in a relationship.

A good way to measure the difference between an occasional struggle and ED is the percentage of times getting an erection is a problem. If the struggle to obtain an erection is less than 20 percent of the time, ED is not a concern; however, if the struggle is more than half the time sexual activity is engaged in, action needs to be taken.

What Causes ED?

Erectile dysfunction is a sign something else is wrong. What you may not know but will make complete sense when you stop to think about it is: The same factors that cause you to be overweight, obese, or have high cholesterol, hypertension, diabetes, or cardiovascular disease are the same factors that cause erectile dysfunction.

Hardened arteries are a good example. The penis depends upon blood flow to function properly, just like any other part of the body; therefore, when its blood supply is blocked or compromised, there is no way to achieve an erection. The penis also depends upon nerve impulses to achieve an erection. If the nerves are not working correctly due to a stroke or diabetes, an erection is not possible.

Certain surgeries, those usually related to living an inflammatory lifestyle like colon cancer surgery, can also contribute to ED.

The hormonal imbalance and chronic inflammation that lead to erectile dysfunction may be due to a number of lifestyle factors, including:

- **Consuming the Western Un-Natural Food Diet**
- **Indulging in alcohol, tobacco use, and prescription drugs**

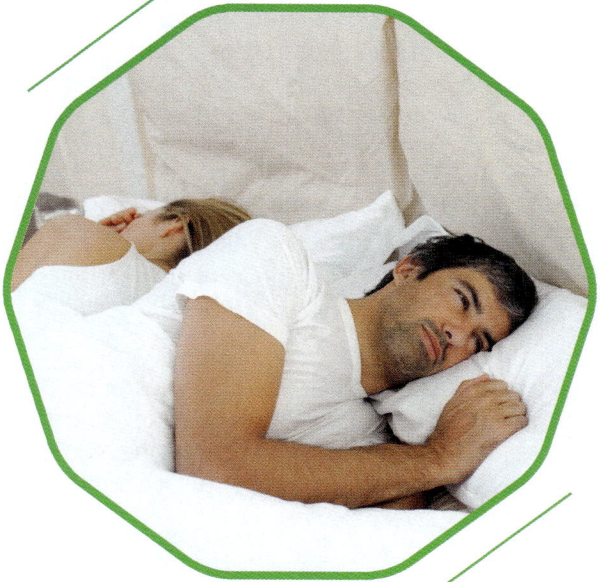

Treatments (Consider as a Very Last Resort)

The options to treat ED include:

- **Drugs** - May come with the side effects of indigestion, nasal congestion, flushing, headaches, and temporary visual disturbance.
- **Invasive Surgery** - Such as a penile implant.
- **Hormone Therapy** - With side effects.
- **Mechanical Devices** - Such as penile constriction rings, which may be uncomfortable and embarrassing.
- **Injection Therapy into the Penis** - Can be painful and leave scarring; may also cause dizziness, hypertension, and even lead to a prolonged, painful erection.

An uncommon condition called Peyronie's disease may also lead to ED. This is a painful condition in which a man's penis, because of damage from an accident or possibly an immune system disorder, develops scar tissue, leading to a curve during an erection.

Erectile Dysfunction in Men: Are Stress and Anxiety to Blame?

Stress and self-doubt can cause occasional difficulties in the bedroom. However, long-term stress and chronic anxiety can be significant contributing factors in the struggle with ED. With constant pressure from work and family, it's no wonder that an estimated 15 to 30 million men have ED.

According to the Weill Cornell Medical College James Buchanan Brady Foundation Department of Urology, the stress and ED connection is clear. Psychological triggers for erectile dysfunction may include stress and anxiety related to personal, financial, or marital problems.

Cornell Urology explains, "For example, a sexually active man may suddenly find himself unable to have an erection shortly after losing his job. It is possible for the man's stress and anxiety to interfere with nerve impulses from his brain when he attempts sexual intercourse."

> ♂ *"Performance anxiety" is an ED explanation you may hear often in the bedroom.*

Once a man has difficulty achieving an erection and feels he cannot perform, it triggers even more anxiety. Lahey Clinic urologist and erectile dysfunction expert Nelson E. Bennett, M.D., takes it a step further. Dr. Bennett explains that ED may also stem from issues in a relationship, whether performance anxiety in a new relationship or loss of desire that creates anxiety in a long-term relationship.

Dr. Bennett says, "These problems can build, and temporary sexual issues can become real erectile dysfunction problems."

Based on 2003 research published in the *International Journal of Impotence Research*, anxiety that contributes to ED may be more of a problem than men have been led to believe. Anxiety can play a major role in issues linked to erectile dysfunction. The psychological and behavioral effects of ED, such as distance, conflict, and uneasiness, will in turn create a vicious cycle that makes it even more difficult to have a healthy sex life.

If your stress and anxiety have triggered ED, it is important to address the root of the issue first of all. Counseling, exercise, lifestyle changes, and the nutritional therapy outlined in this book can all be used to ease stress and anxiety, naturally.

Stress and anxiety can creep in and affect every part of your life. If your sex life has been compromised by chronic stress, the answer does not come in a prescription pill for ED or anxiety. In order to treat ED, you must see the big picture. Eliminating top triggers like stress and anxiety can naturally improve sexual health.

Sources: Cornell Urology
EverydayHealth.com
International Journal of Impotence Research (2003) 15, Suppl 2, S16–S19. doi:10.1038/sj.ijir.3900994

Recommended Products for Stress and Anxiety in Men

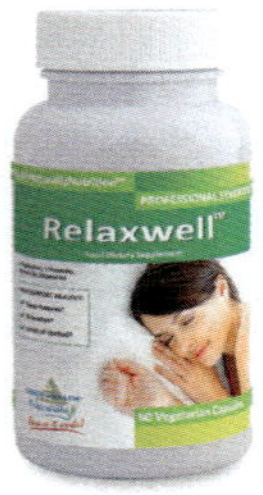

Relaxwell - Professional Strength Super Nutrient Formula

Take Relaxwell to combat stress and restlessness during times of high physical and mental demand, or make Relaxwell part of your daily supplementation to always be well rested and ready for anything that comes your way.

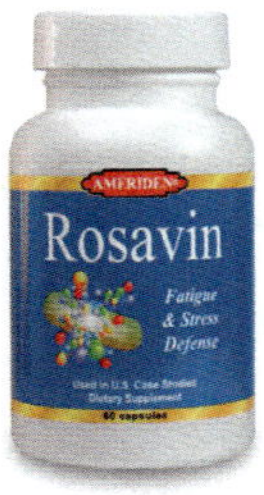

Rosavin - Powerful Fatigue and Stress Defense

Siberian Rhodiola Rosea is purported to provide potential adaptogenic responses to a number of environmental stressors. This action may help the body to fight mood swings, enhance memory and mental performance, assist in maintaining energy levels and stamina, increase circulation in the brain, and aid weight management.

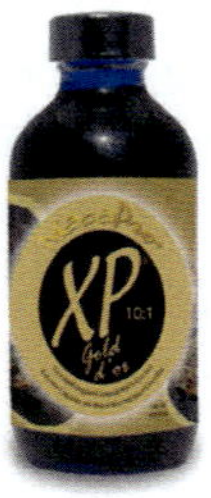

MacaPro XP Gold Liquid

Maca is a root that grows in Peru at altitudes of 14,000 feet. A true superfood, Maca root contains calcium, magnesium, phosphorous, iron, other essential vitamins and minerals, and 19 amino acids. It has been traditionally used as an adaptogen and as a nutritious food to provide optimal wellbeing.

Hormonal Imbalances

The medical dictionary tells us that hormones are chemical substances produced in the body, which have a specific regulatory effect on the activity of certain cells or a certain organ or organs.

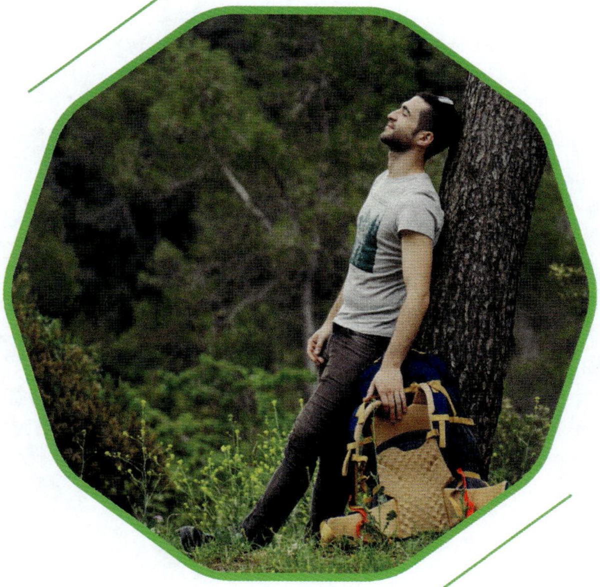

What About Male Hormones?

Even though there is not as much discussion about men and their hormones, these chemical substances are just as crucial to a man's health as they are to a woman's health. The concerns discussed in this book are related to hormonal imbalances. There is much controversy over male hormone replacement, just as there is over female hormone replacement. This is due to the inevitable side effects and possible disease brought on by their use.

The men's health concerns discussed here are hormonally dependent—meaning, whether hormones are too high or too low, the survival of the disease or dysfunction depends upon the hormonal imbalance.

♂ Balance cannot be found in a drug, a patch, or an injection. A better way is to find natural balance.

Men have many different kinds of hormones; however, testosterone is the hormone that often needs the most attention. Really Healthy Foods (anti-inflammatory) and high-quality supplements can bring testosterone levels, other hormone levels, and the body back into balance.

Really Healthy Foods are higher in antioxidants, the substances that fight off and neutralize free radicals. Merely existing creates free radicals, as does exercise and the process of eating and digestion. We do require some level of free radicals to function; however, due to our excessive lifestyles of drinking, smoking, and eating toxic foods, our bodies are in overload.

Fortunately, antioxidants available in high-quality foods and supplements can fight off these free radicals and the damage they do to the body. This includes the inflammation associated with men's health issues.

The Western Un-Natural Food Diet

Nutritional therapy comes in the form of an anti-inflammatory diet and the appropriate supplementation. These components are crucial in strengthening the immune system, decreasing inflammation, and winning the battle against prostate cancer—as well as BPH and prostatitis. Keep in mind, these conditions stem from inflammation too.

Over a third of the cancer deaths every year in Western countries can be attributed to diet alone. The World Health Organization says that at least one third of all cancer cases are preventable. Certain cancers, including prostate cancer, are up to 80 percent attributable to diet. Imagine the impact that could be made in the fight against prostate cancer if nutritional therapy was embraced and other cancer-promoting lifestyle habits were addressed.

> ♂ *An anti-inflammatory diet is essential when dealing with chronic inflammation.*

A diet which will definitely hinder one's recovery from men's health issues is the Western Un-Natural Food Diet. Nothing affects us more than what we choose to eat at least three to four times a day, every day. Most of us lack the essential nutrients in our diet needed for good health, spreading inflammation. This absence of nutrients combined with one or several other unhealthy lifestyle choices can perpetuate the diseases and health issues more common in men.

The "Balanced Western Diet" (now better described as the Western Un-Natural Food Diet) is the number one disease-promoting and inflammation-producing diet in modern society. It is consumed more and more on a daily basis.

This highly inflammatory diet is made up of sugary foods in the form of breads, pastas, cereals, and potatoes. The Western Un-Natural Food Diet is way too high in unhealthy fats and lacks the antioxidants and phytochemicals that are crucial for eliminating free radicals. This all too common diet is lacking in high-fiber foods and the foods that provide essential nutrients necessary to find relief from men's health issues.

These missing foods, recommended especially for prostate cancer, include:

- **Allium Vegetables** - Onions, leeks, scallions, and garlic
- **Beans** - Except when temporarily contraindicated for recovery
- **Cruciferous Vegetables** - Cabbage, cauliflower, and broccoli
- **Dark-Skinned Fruits and Vegetables** - Especially those high in lycopene (bright red foods, e.g., tomatoes)
- **Nuts**
- **Seeds**

A number of nutritionally sound physicians now call the ketogenic diet the first course of cancer treatment after diagnosis. The ketogenic diet is a high-fat, low-carbohydrate diet that starves cancer cells of their primary food source: sugar. Cancer cells only feed on glucose. The ketogenic diet encourages cancer cells to starve and die by severely restricting sugar.

Dr. Scheck of the Barrow Neuro-Oncology Research Laboratory confirms the effects of the ketogenic diet when used alongside cancer therapies, like chemotherapy and radiation, to "slow the growth of living cancer cells and significantly increase survival time."

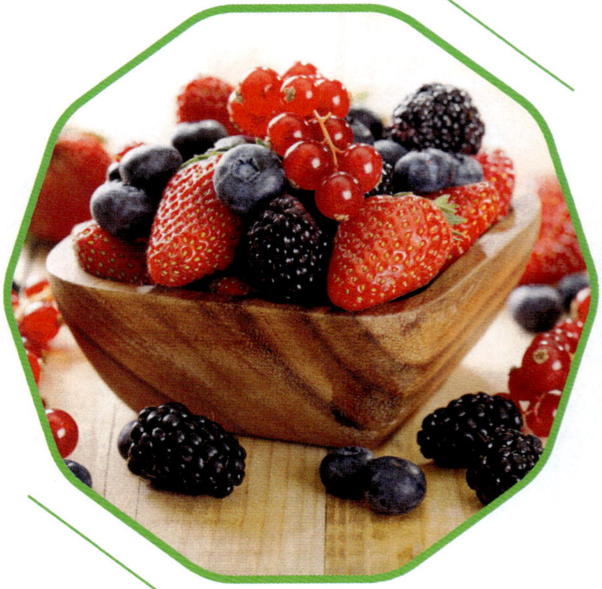

It's Time to Rethink Animal Protein

Unfortunately, what is not missing in the Western Un-Natural Food diet is animal protein. Many of the health concerns in Westernized societies, including chronic disease and cancer, can be traced back to the consumption of animal products (red meat, chicken, fish, milk, and eggs) and animal protein, specifically.

Research conducted across the globe showed an indisputable link between the consumption of animal protein and cancer.

When levels of animal protein consumed in the diet went up, so did cancer rates. All forms of animal protein were studied and showed similar results; however, casein (the protein in dairy) had the strongest effect. Furthermore, studies found that what we eat can actually *manipulate* the gene responsible for cancer by turning it off and on in relation to the amount of animal protein in the diet.

More animal protein, more cancer. The same amounts of vegetable protein showed no such relationship.

If you cut back or eliminate animal protein, will you become protein deficient? Think about this. The time in our lives when we need the most protein is when we are an infant. Human breast milk is only 5 percent protein! The truth is that if you are choosing a variety of healthy plant-based foods, you will provide your body with all the protein it requires.

Glucose in the Bloodstream

The consumption of foods high in sugar, i.e., refined sugars and carbohydrates, causes glucose in the bloodstream to rise very quickly. This in turn signals the body to release insulin and IGF-1. Insulin assists the sugar in entering the cells, and IGF-1 is responsible for stimulating cell growth.

Glucose is the primary type of sugar in the bloodstream and is the main source of energy for the cells in the body. It's obvious we need glucose to live; however, research has shown blood sugar levels that exceed 110 mg/dl increase the risk for cancer. Cancer cells utilize sugar as an energy source too, especially in the absence of oxygen, a scenario far too common in an acidic body.

A high-sugar diet is a cancer-promoting diet. This is why it's crucial to implement a diet that keeps blood sugar levels stable and consistent.

High blood sugar levels and the link to cancer:

- Support the inflammatory process
- Promote cell growth (including cancer cells)
- Foster tumor growth

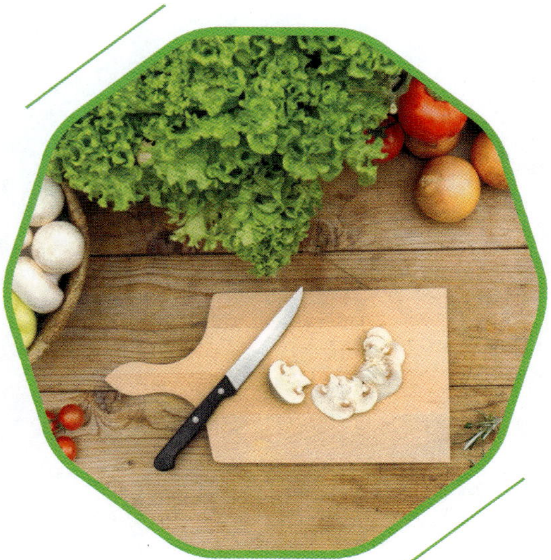

Can I Reverse My Prostate Condition, ED, or Hormonal Imbalance?

I prefer not to use the word "cure" when talking about these health conditions since many cases are directly related to or exacerbated by lifestyle factors.

Cure is a popular medical buzzword, although the medical field cannot provide cures. (Many people argue that this is on purpose since it would put Big Pharma out of business.) Every health condition has a cause. When you take away the underlying cause and follow a non-inflammatory lifestyle, your body will have the support it needs to repair itself, in many cases.

When you remove the cause and support your body with healthy lifestyle choices and nutrients, you can often grow healthy again. You may call this a cure, but I believe it to be making healthy lifestyle choices.

Since these health conditions are inflammatory, a non-inflammatory lifestyle is a must. It's important to stay hydrated by drinking six to eight 16 ounce (500 ml) glasses of pure, clean water per day. You can heal your body with vital nutrients and antioxidants found in vitamins, minerals, healthy carbohydrates, amino acids, and essential fatty acids.

Optimal Nutritional Management

Optimal nutritional management is essential for the repair of damaged tissues, the reduction of inflammation, and for the quality, as well as the length, of life.

Did you know those who consider themselves happy have less inflammation than those who don't? It could certainly be argued that a well-rested, hormonally balanced man who is of a healthy weight; limits toxins; focuses on a diet bountiful in foods which are nourishing, anti-inflammatory, and a source of enzymes and antioxidants; and who also supplements with high-quality nutrients is an individual who is happy indeed!

Nutritional therapy supports healing.

The initial detox can be uncomfortable but only temporarily.

Eating right can minimize the effects.

. . . regenerate with healthy lifestyle and nutrients . . .

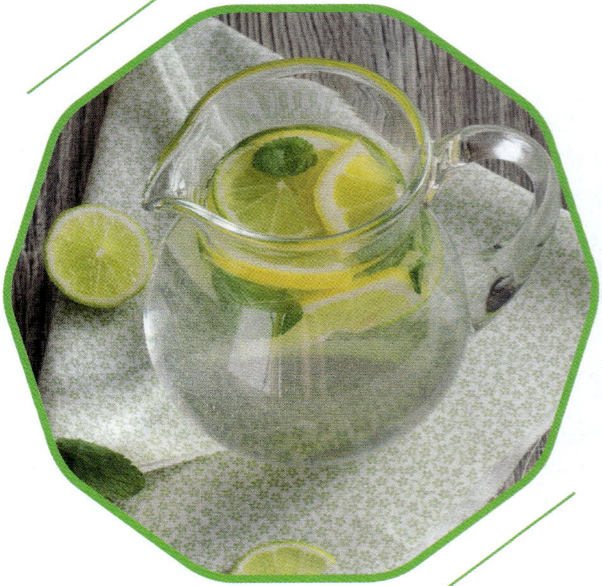

The Nutrients You Need

According to research, these nutrients can manage or prevent men's health issues, in most cases:

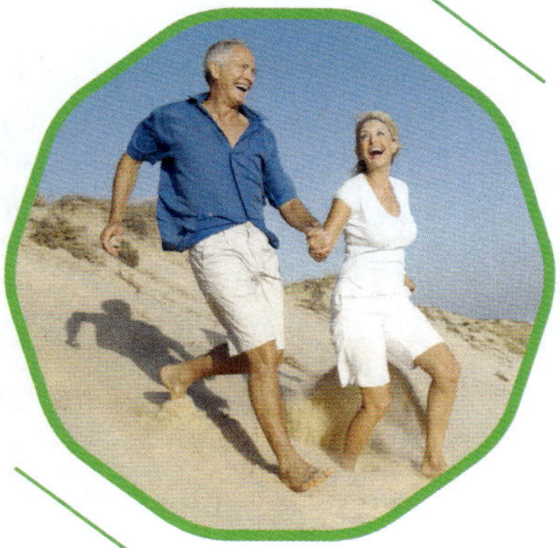

- **Vitamins A, B2, B6, D3, E, Copper, Pomegranate Powder Extract, Selenium, and Zinc** - Designed to support prostate maintenance and overall health, along with Saw Palmetto Extract, Nettle Root Extract, Uva Ursi Extract, L-Glycine, L-Alanine, Lycored Beadlets, Panax Ginseng Extract, and a Proprietary Blend.

- **Curcuminx4000 (from Meriva® curcuma longa extract), Ecklonia Cava Extract 25:1, Serrapeptase, and Vitamin D3** - Provide relief from inflammation.

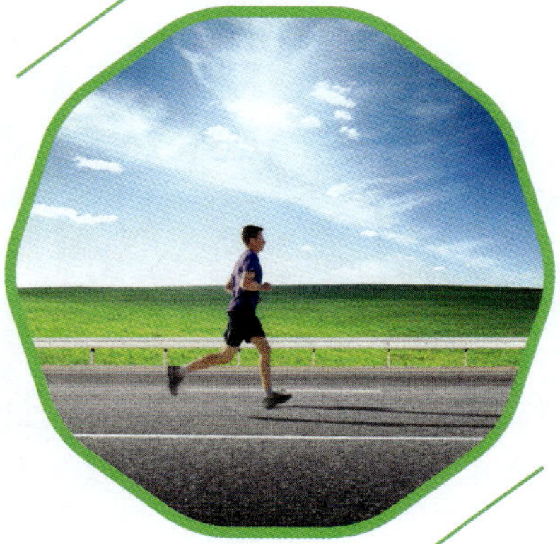

- **Iodine (in its atomic form)** - Essential for a completely healthy body.

- **29 Probiotic Microflora "Soil-Based-Organisms" (SBOs)** - Support the gut and immune system, promoting normal bowel function. Contains Calcium, Chromium, Copper, Folic Acid, Inositol, Magnesium, Concentrate Ionic Trace Minerals, Manganese, Organic Seleniumethionine, Potassium, Zinc, Phosphorous, Biotin, Iodine, Boron, Molybdenum, Chloride Concentrate, Amino Acid Complex, Aloe Vera Extract (200:1), and Vitamins A, B1, B12, B2, B3, B5, B6, C, D, E, and K.

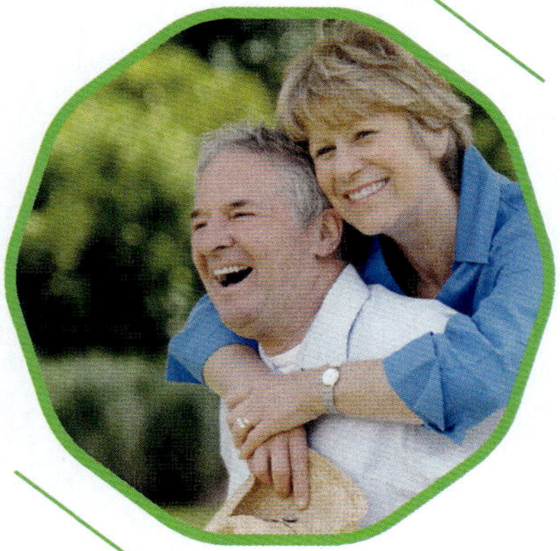

- **Sodium Thiocyanate and Sodium Hypothiocyanate** - Contain thiocyanates that can help to clear any infections that may reside in the cells.

What If My Doctor Doesn't Support My Recovery?

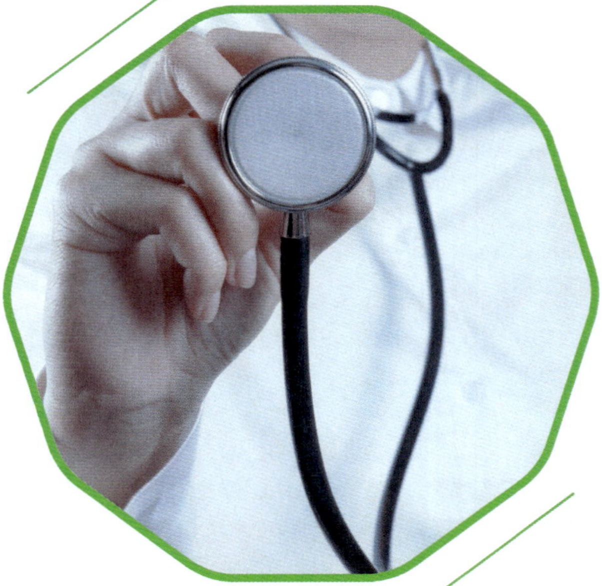

You can use the Men's Health Rehabilitation Program to improve your health! Your doctor has an obligation to stick with the prescription drug outline that fits into the pharmaceutical industry monopoly. This includes the AMA in the US and the GMC in the UK.

Make no mistake - these organizations make money off basic healthcare for sick individuals. They don't have a business model that promotes actual health recovery in any way, shape, or form. These organizations push a patented prescription drug protocol that allows them to charge outrageous prices for drug use over a lifetime. At the very best, these drugs may help the patient to feel better, but in many scenarios, they could lead to their death.

♂ These industries won't support long-term health recovery in any circumstance!

These organizations are protected by the FDA in the US and the MHRA in the UK. They receive backing from powerful political parties that continue to fund the disease-promoting monopoly I have just described.

Yet when you follow the Men's Health Rehabilitation Program to the letter, you can see results within 30 days.

Your Men's Health Rehabilitation Plan

10 Steps for Long-Term Health Recovery

This self-recovery protocol can be used by sufferers of men's health issues, in most cases:

1 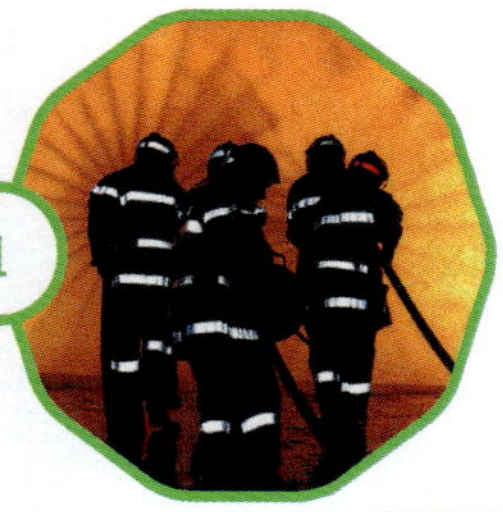 Clear inflammation and facilitate healing

2 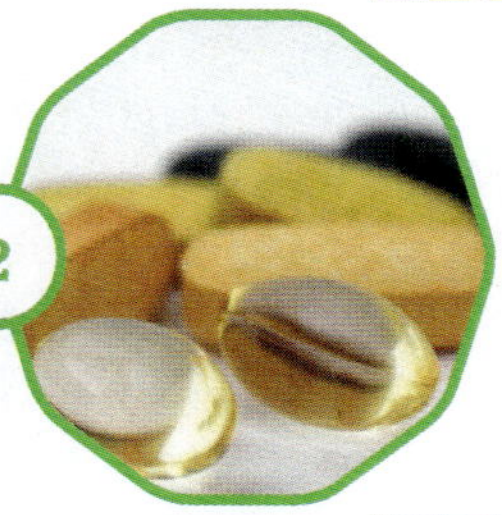 Supplement missing nutrients

3 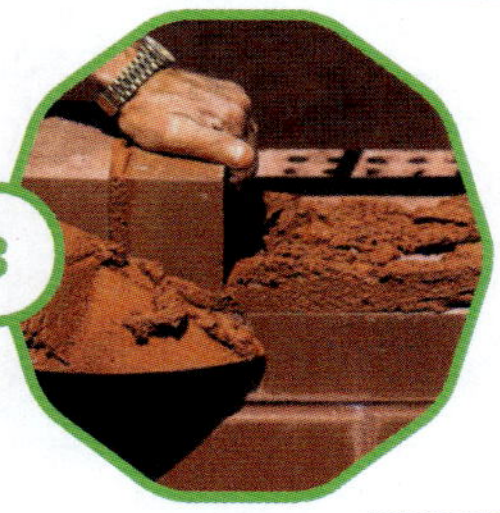 Boost the immune system

4 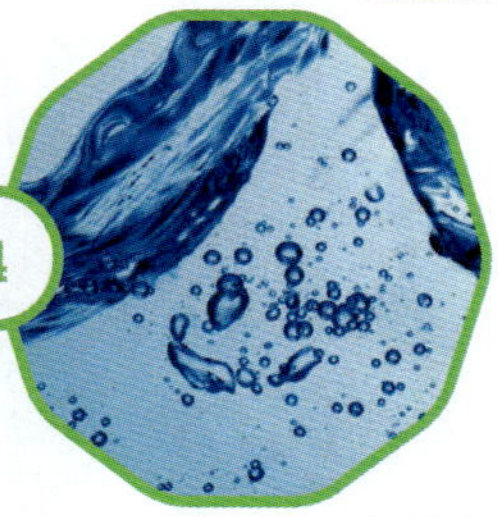 Drink more water

5 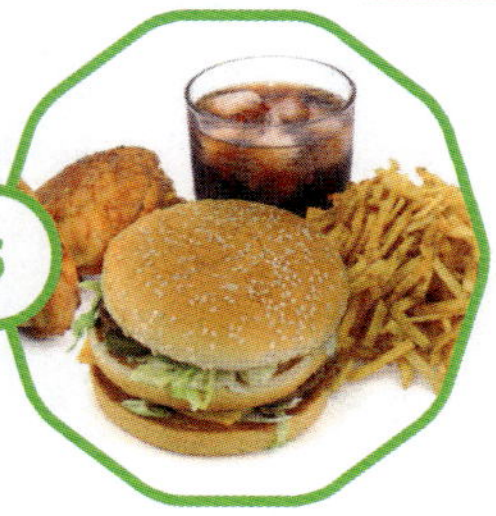 Cut out unnatural foods

6 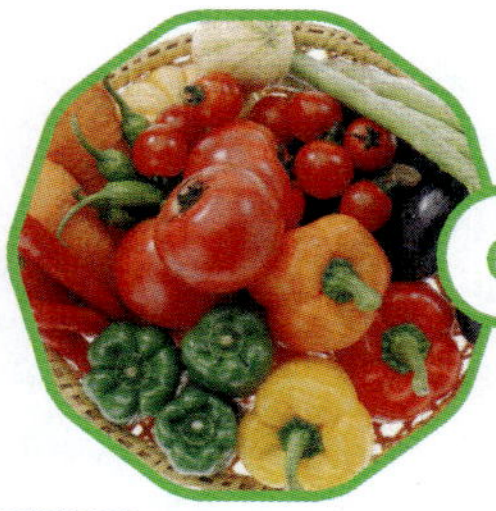 Eat really healthy foods

7 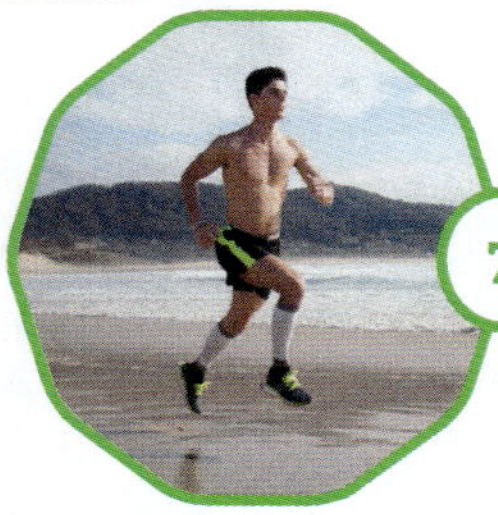 Stay active daily

8 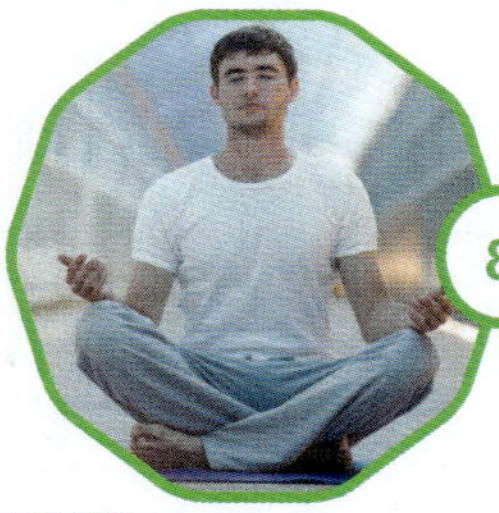 Learn proper breathing

9 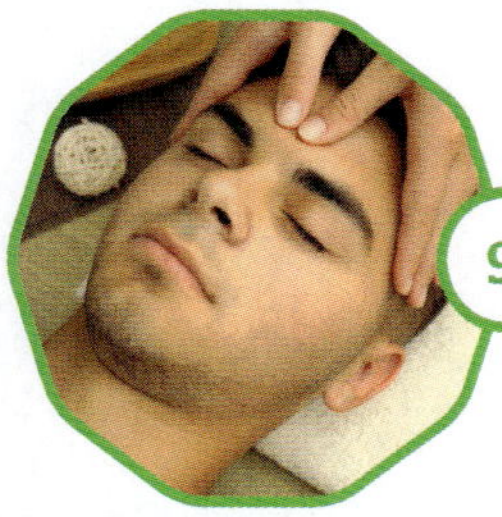 Stimulate acupressure points

10 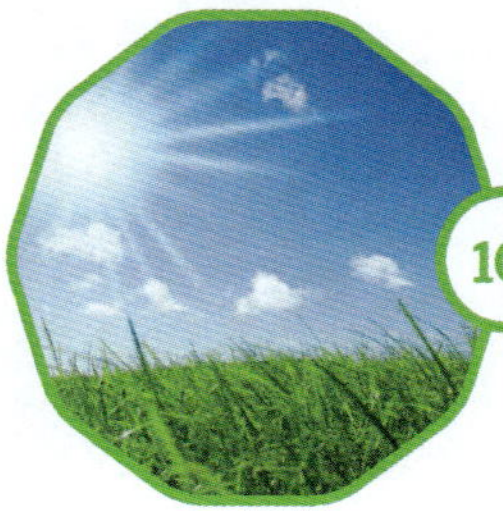 Get more sun exposure

It's almost impossible *not* to see significant health changes after applying many of the points in this 10 Step Plan. You can clear up numerous symptoms and may see a full recovery, in many cases.

For details of the following suggested formulas, turn to **page 37.**

1. Clear Inflammation and Facilitate Healing

Basic Plan

- **Prostate Plus+** - Designed for prostate maintenance and health. Take 2 capsules daily.

- **Serranol** - Provides relief for pain and inflammation. Take 2 capsules x 3 times per day. Take 30 minutes before eating a meal with water. Reduce to 1 x 3 after a good relief.

- **Nascent Iodine Drops** - Iodine is essential for a completely healthy body. Take 5 drops x 3 times per day in 20ml of water; swish around the mouth for 30 seconds before swallowing. Build over 2 weeks to 15 x 3 until well and then slowly reduce back to 5 x 3. Take first dose on waking, second midmorning, and third midafternoon. Note that iodine needs a supplement containing selenium to activate it, such as Active Life, D.I.P. Daily Immune Protection, or B4 Health Spray.

2. Supplement Missing Nutrients

Advanced Plan

- **Prostate Plus+** - Designed for prostate maintenance and health. Take 2 capsules daily.

- **Serranol** - Provides relief for pain and inflammation. Take 2 capsules x 3 times per day. Take 30 minutes before eating a meal with water. Reduce to 1 x 3 after a good relief.

- **Nascent Iodine Drops** - Iodine is essential for a completely healthy body. Take 5 drops x 3 times per day in 20ml of water; swish around the mouth for 30 seconds before swallowing. Build over 2 weeks to 15 x 3 until well and then slowly reduce back to 5 x 3. Take first dose on waking, second midmorning, and third midafternoon. Note that iodine needs a supplement containing selenium to activate it, such as Active Life, D.I.P. Daily Immune Protection, or B4 Health Spray.

- **Prescript-Assist** – Soil-based probiotic supports the gut immune system and promotes normal bowel function. Take 1 capsule x 2 times per day. You will likely need to take this therapeutically and then for maintenance.

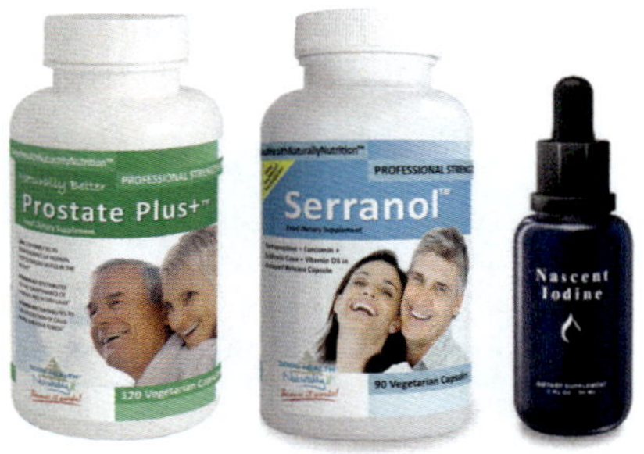

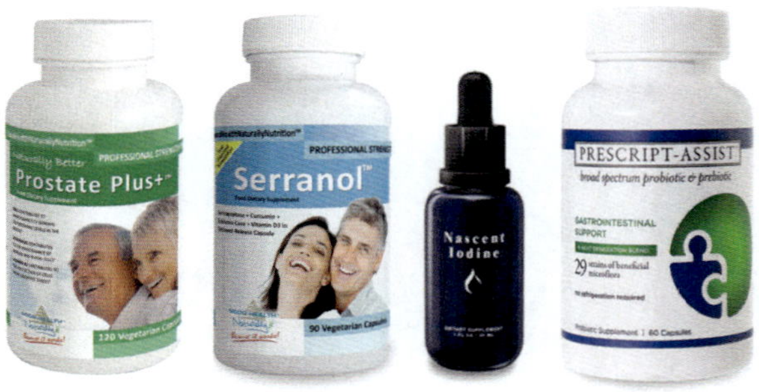

3. Boost the Immune System

Ultimate Plan

- **Prostate Plus+** - Designed for prostate maintenance and health. Take 2 capsules daily.
- **Serranol** - Provides relief for pain and inflammation. Take 2 capsules x 3 times per day. Take 30 minutes before eating a meal with water. Reduce to 1 x 3 after a good relief.
- **Nascent Iodine Drops** - Iodine is essential for a completely healthy body. Take 5 drops x 3 times per day in 20ml of water; swish around the mouth for 30 seconds before swallowing. Build over 2 weeks to 15 x 3 until well and then slowly reduce back to 5 x 3. Take first dose on waking, second midmorning, and third midafternoon. Note that iodine needs a supplement containing selenium to activate it, such as Active Life, D.I.P. Daily Immune Protection, or B4 Health Spray.
- **Prescript-Assist** – Soil-based probiotic supports the gut immune system and promotes normal bowel function. Take 1 capsule x 2 times per day. You will likely need to take this therapeutically and then for maintenance.
- **Active Life** - Delivers a full spectrum of 90 liquid, highly-absorbable multivitamins and minerals. Take 15ml x 2 times daily with meals.

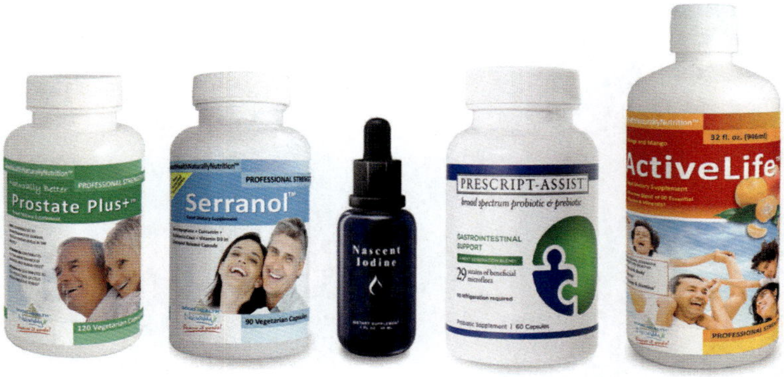

Optional - But Highly Recommended for At Least 1 to 2 Months

- **1st Line Immune Support Kit** - Clears any infection that may reside in the cells. Always take at least 90 minutes before food and 90 minutes after food. Take 1 kit daily for 3 days (total of 3). *Three kits should be taken as a minimum; in serious conditions, 10 kits are better if finances allow.*

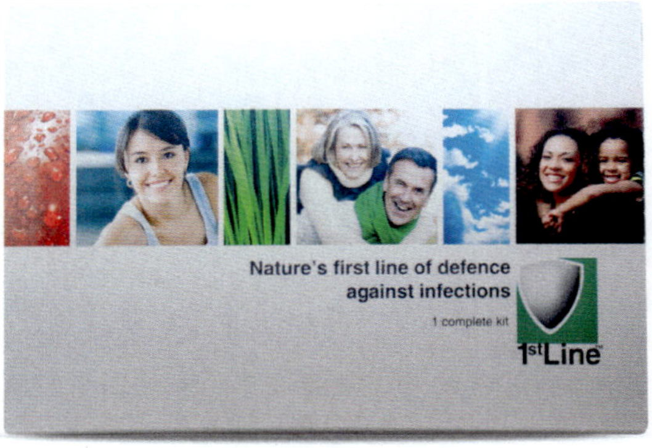

4. Drink More Water

Drink at least 6-8 glasses of RO filtered or distilled water each day; add a generous pinch of baking soda to each glass. This step is essential for internal organ support.

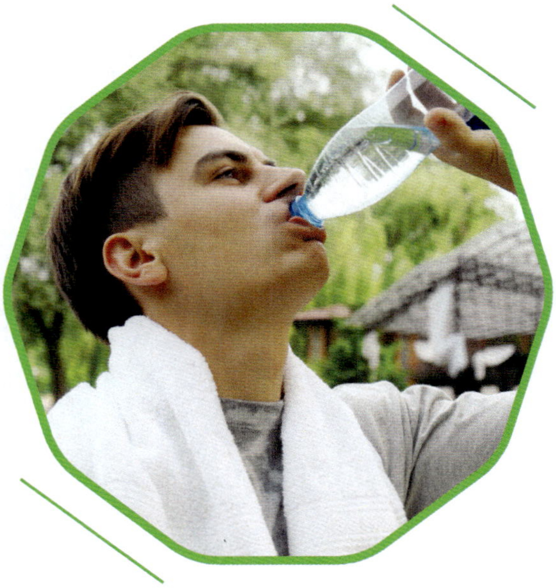

5. Cut Out Unnatural Foods

Until you've achieved full recovery, cut out starchy carbohydrates altogether, i.e. pastries, cookies, breads, breakfast cereals, pasta, and potatoes, as well as processed foods and milk products.

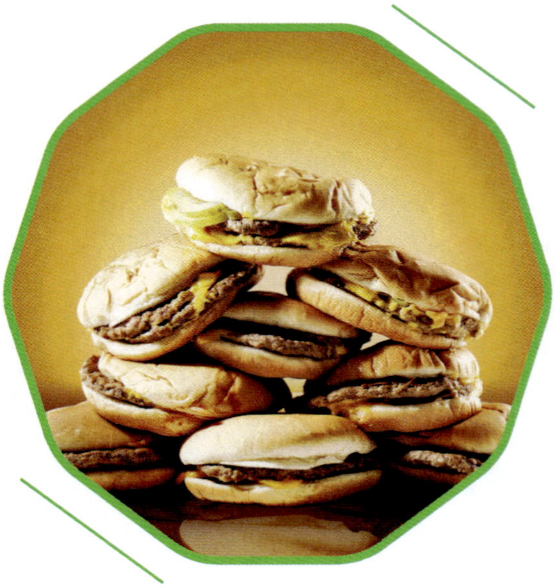

Note: Don't eat turnips, parsnips, and rice, except for small portions of wild rice, brown rice, and sweet potatoes/yams.

6. Eat Really Healthy Foods.

Make sure to eat some of these foods every two hours for the first few months of recovery:

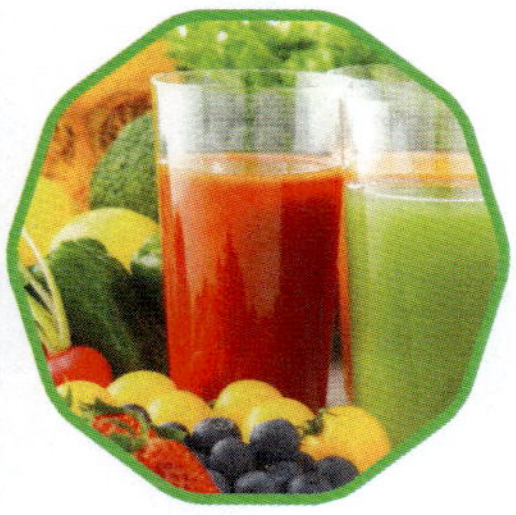

Eat 9-14 servings of fresh or frozen vegetables each day: Try them in soups, steamed, stir-fried, juiced, etc. Eat 50 percent raw, juiced vegetables (preferably organic) and use the pulp to make soup. Blended veggies promote easier digestion.

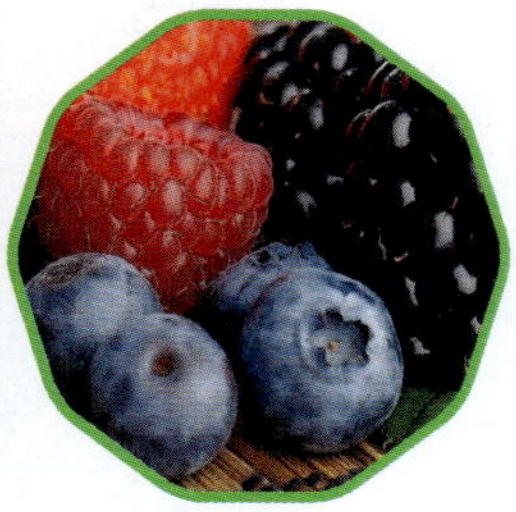

Eat 5 servings of dark-skinned fruits (like cherries, red grapes, blueberries, etc.) that are rich in antioxidants each day.

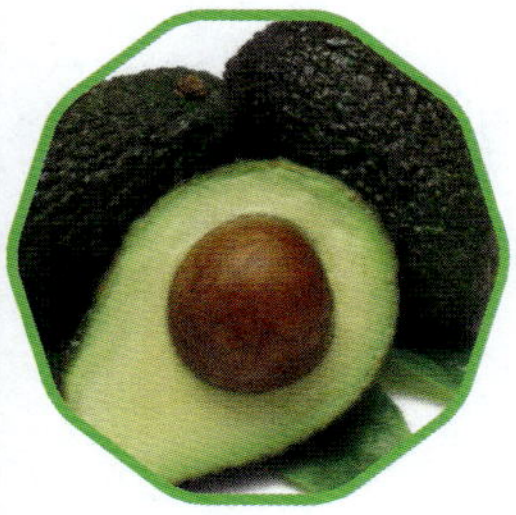

Remember that avocados are a number one superfood with almost a complete spectrum of nutrients. If they are readily available in your area, try to eat at least two a day to promote health recovery. Avocados support men's health, heart disease, diabetes, and even cancer rehabilitation.

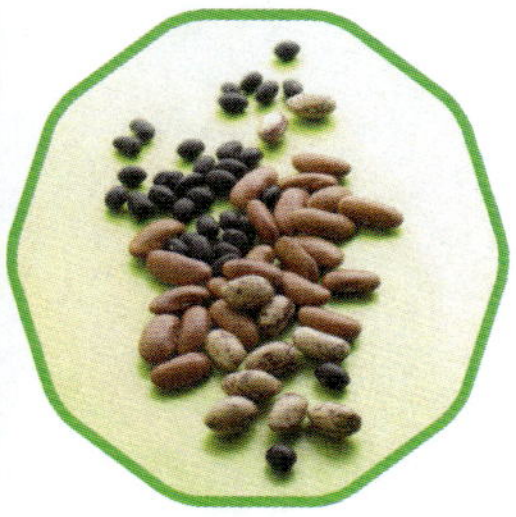

Eat 5 servings of nuts, beans, and seeds (soaked, mashed nuts and seeds).

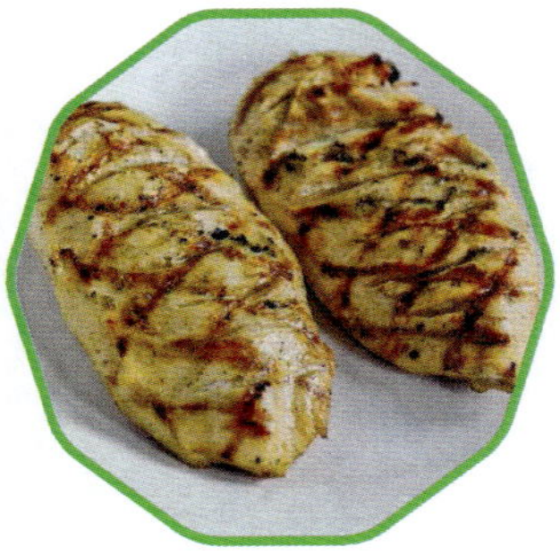

Eat pasture-fed chicken and other meats, only a few servings per week. Grass-fed meat is recommended above corn or grain-fed meat sources.

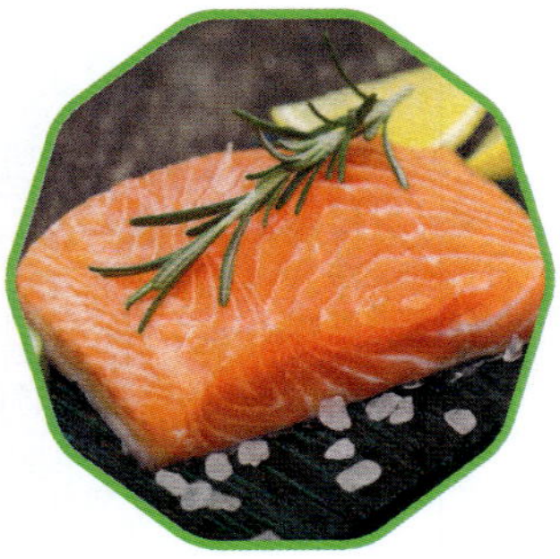

Eat a minimum of 3-4 servings of oily fish each week, if you eat fish. Choose a variety of healthy fish like mackerel, sardines, salmon, etc. Canned fish is a nutritious option, although wild caught fish is recommended.

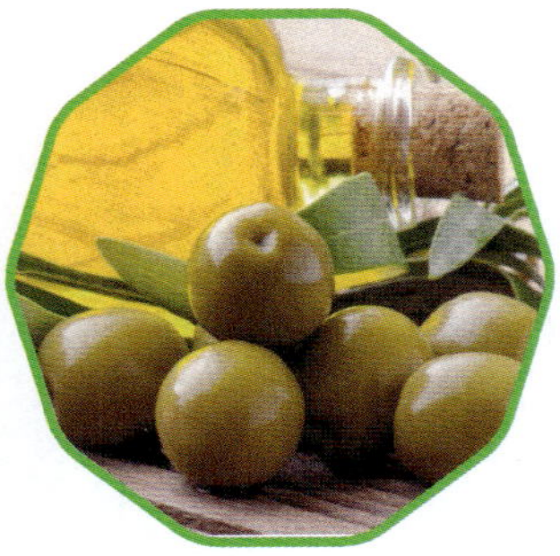

Add healthy oils to your favorite foods, like krill, omega 3, hemp, coconut, and olive oils. Pair with healthy carbohydrate alternatives, like amaranth, quinoa, buckwheat, and chai and millet seeds. You can also try couscous, if you aren't allergic to gluten protein (celiac disease).

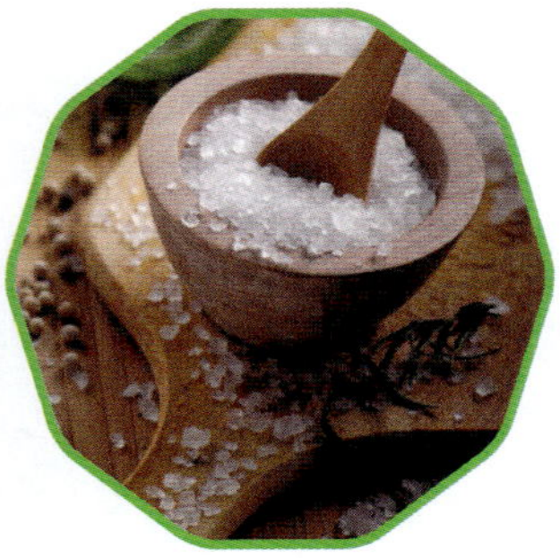

Add 3-5 teaspoons of sea or rock salt, depending on the heat and your body mass, to water or food each day. Remember that sea or rock salt does not contain the important mineral iodine, so Nascent Iodine is included in your Rehabilitation Plan.

Recommended Vegetables

Note: Vegetables may not be available in all countries.

- Artichoke
- Asian Vegetable Sprouts (Wheat, Barley, Alfalfa, etc.)
- Asparagus
- Avocado
- Beetroot
- Broad Beans
- Broccoli
- Brussel Sprouts
- Cabbage (Various Types)
- Capsicum
- Carrots
- Cauliflower
- Celeriac
- Choko
- Cucumber
- Dandelion Leaves
- Dried Peas
- Eggplant (Aubergine)
- Fennel
- Garden Peas
- Garlic
- Kale
- Kohlrabi
- Kumara
- Lettuce (Kos and Various Types)
- Mangetout Peas
- Mushrooms
- Okra
- Onions (Red and White)
- Petit Pois Peas
- Radishes
- Runner Beans
- Seaweed - All Types (Kelp, Wakame, Noni, etc.)
- Silver Beet
- Spinach
- Squash
- Sugar Snap Peas
- Zucchini (Courgettes)

Recommended Fruits

Note: Fruits may not be available in all countries.

- Apple
- Apricot
- Avocado
- Bilberries
- Blackberries
- Blackcurrants
- Blueberries
- Cherimoya
- Cherries
- Damsons
- Dates
- Durian
- Figs
- Gooseberries
- Grapefruit
- Grapes
- Kiwi Fruit
- Limes
- Lychees
- Mango
- Nectarine
- Orange
- Pear
- Pineapple
- Plum/Prune (Dried Plum)
- Pomegranate
- Rambutan
- Raspberries
- Salal Berry
- Satsuma
- Strawberries
- Tangerine
- Western Raspberry (Blackcap)

Healthy Food Pyramid:
Garden of Eden

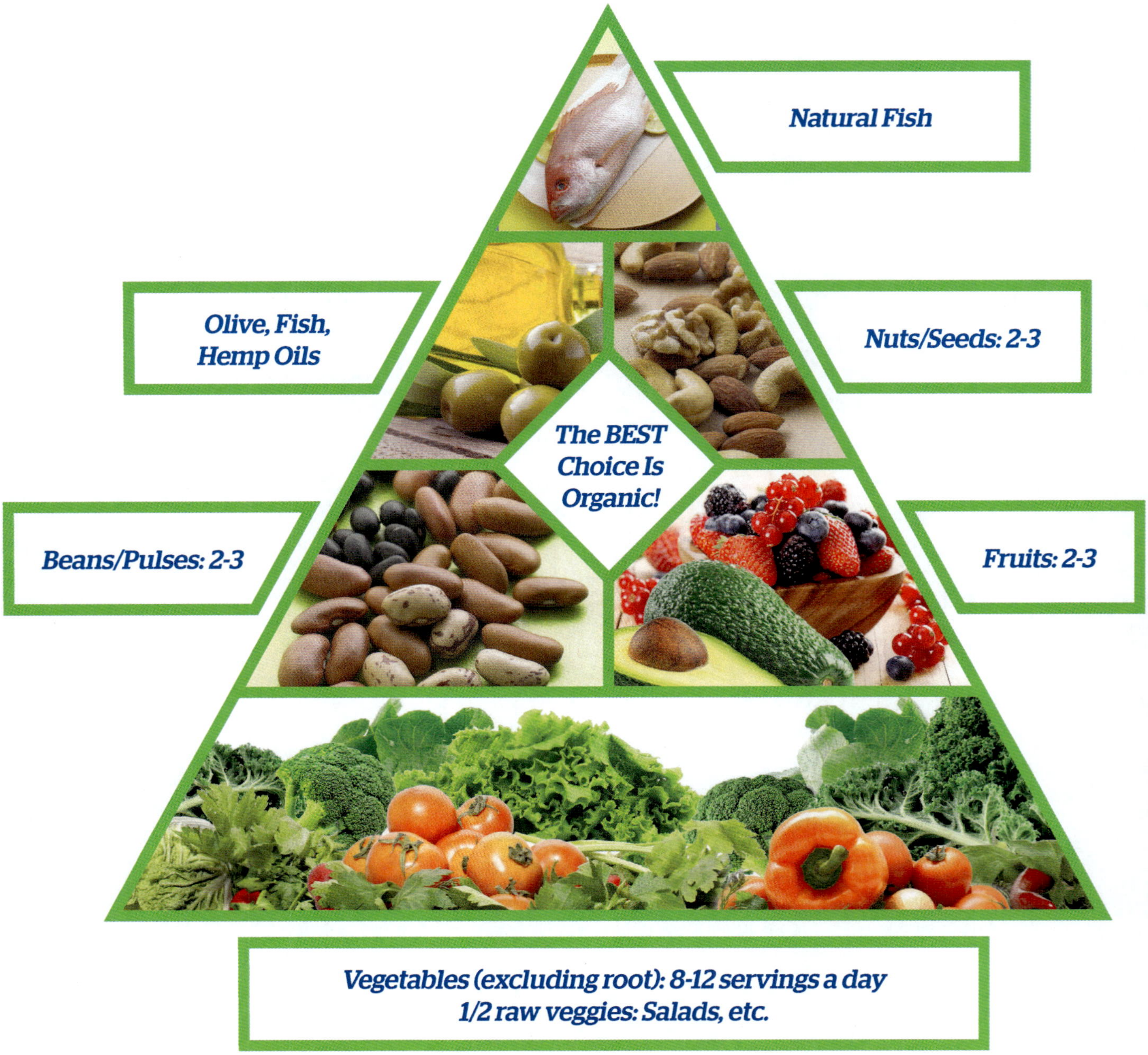

7. Stay Active Daily

Contrary to the opinion of fitness fanatics, there are two simple ways to get your body working better and stronger. And no, they do not include swimming and cycling, although you can add these later if you want to.

One of the two simple ways to exercise is to build up to walking 3-5 miles per day, in a fast, purposely strong way with as long a stride as you can. Keep your hands moving from chest level to belt level as you move with each stride.

Use weights or wrist weights as you improve.

If this is difficult for you at the start, and your lungs are weak, then lie down to exercise to make it easier.

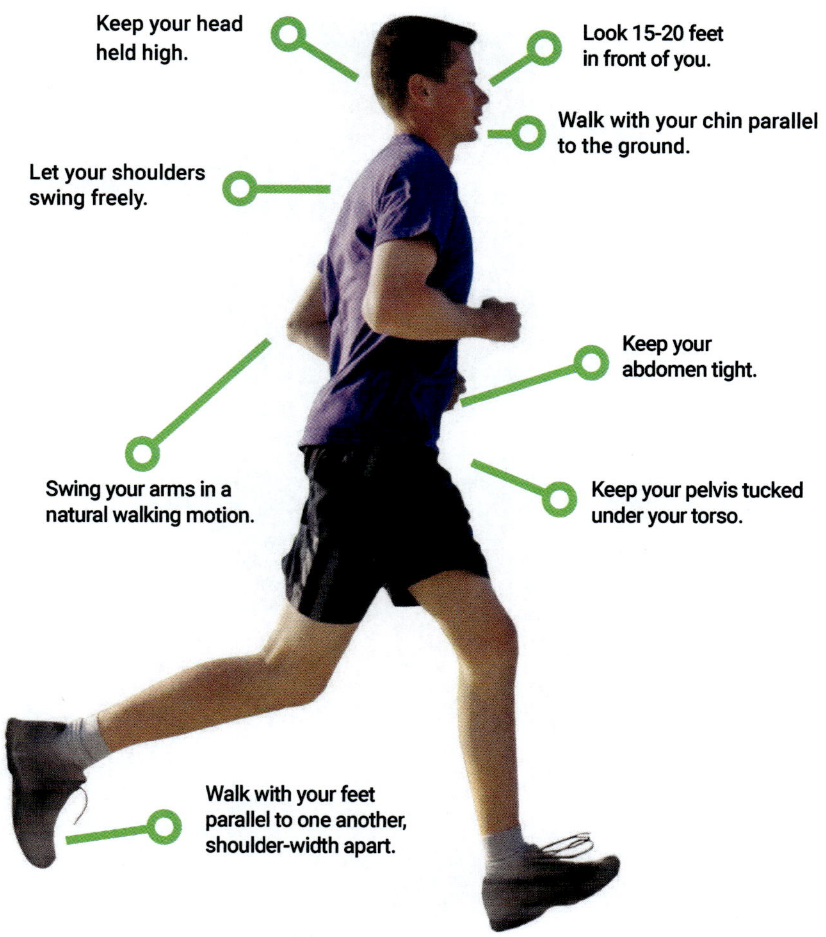

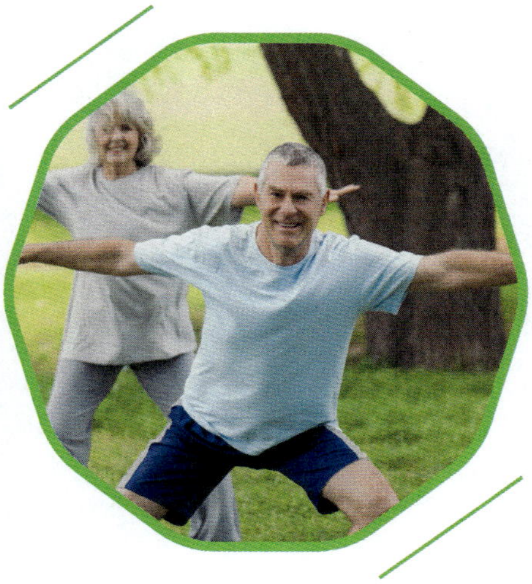

Lie down in a comfortable place. On your bed (if it's firm enough) when you first wake up is a great time and place for this. Bring a knee up to your chest as high as you can get it and then alternate with the other knee. Do as many of these as you can while keeping count. Do this every day and set yourself targets to increase the speed and the number as the weeks go by. You should be doing enough to make your lungs and heart beat faster. At the same time, as you improve your count on your back you need to start your walking and build this up.

The second great exercise for strengthening your lungs is to build up slowly where you can exercise at maximum rate for 2 minutes, 6 times per day. It does not matter what exercise you do, e.g. skipping, star jumps, running on the spot; just about anything works, as long as your heart and lungs are working at maximum capacity. By working at maximum rate, your muscles connected with your heart and lungs will get stronger, and health will balance perfectly.

Movement is a vital part of your recovery plan.

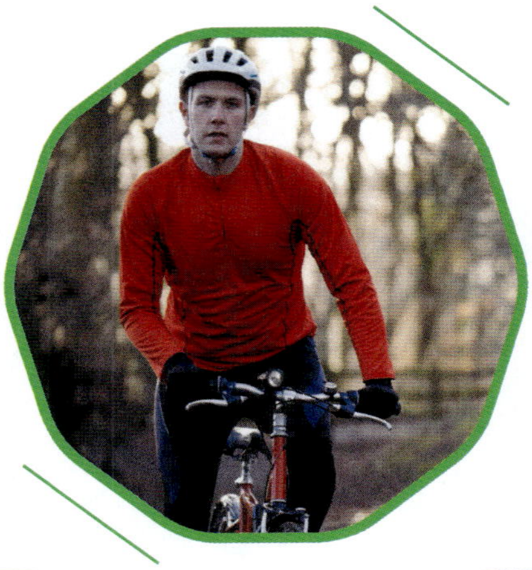

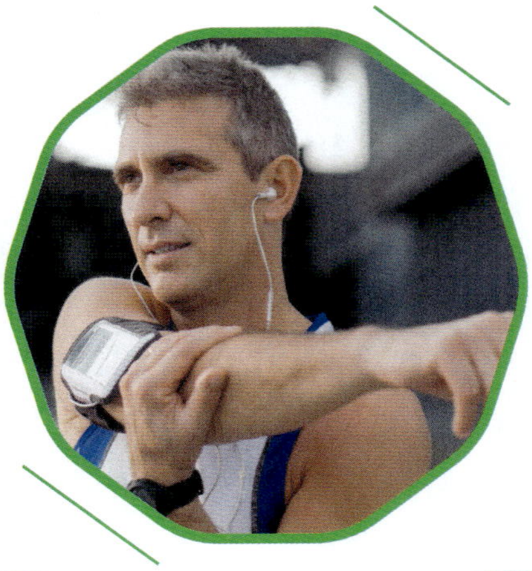

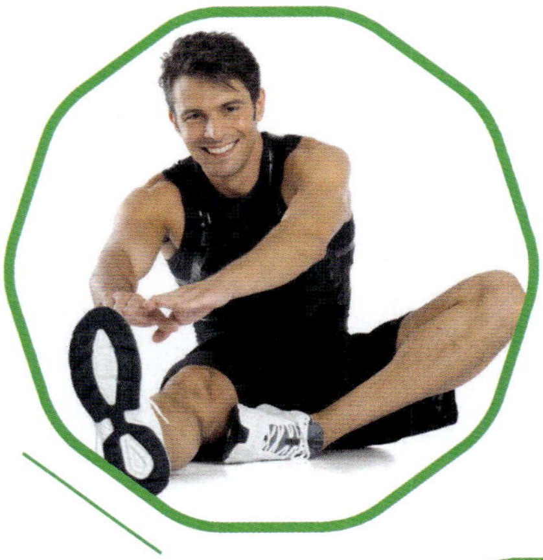

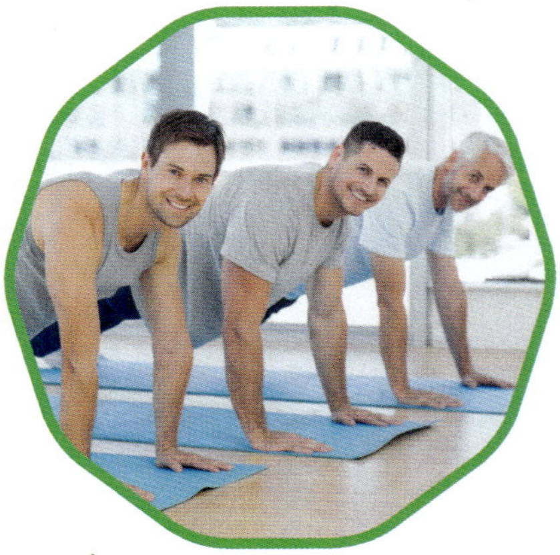

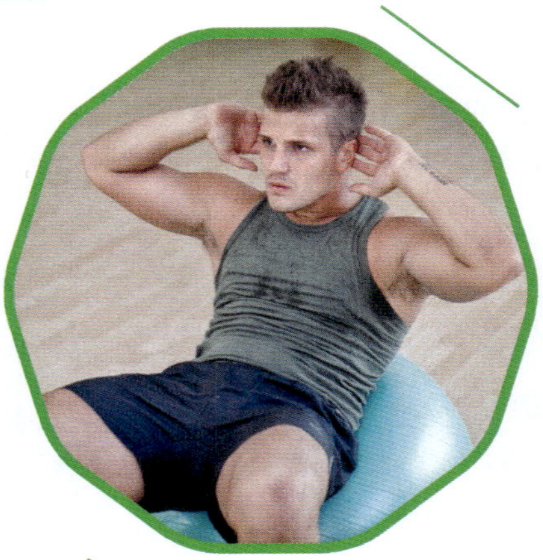

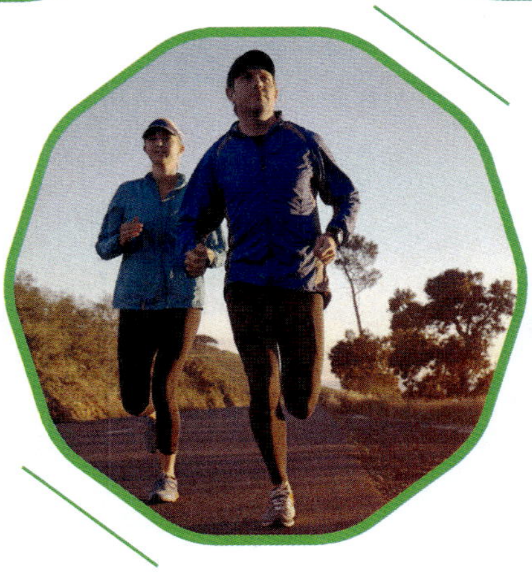

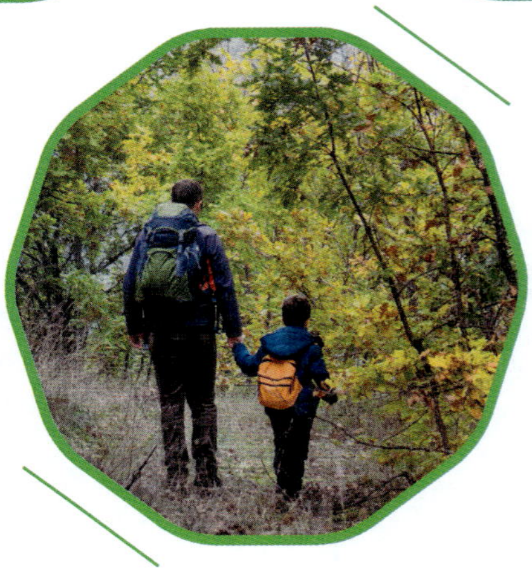

8. Learn Proper Breathing

♂ Breathing properly is critical since oxygen is the foundation of overall health.

There are two types of breathing:

1. **Anxious Breathing:** In the chest.
2. **Relaxed Breathing:** In the diaphragm or stomach area.

The first type of breathing in the chest is related to a stress response and includes hormones like cortisol. This stressful breathing should only be temporary since it is related to a fight-or-flight response that causes hormones to release to relax breathing. If stressful breathing grows chronic, the body will retain carbon dioxide and cortisol to affect healthy functioning systems. Stress breathing will also cause the immune system to weaken, leaving it susceptible to infection.

Make it your number one goal to retrain your body to breathe in a relaxed, healthy manner. This will clear out carbon dioxide and cortisol. When carbon dioxide builds up in your bloodstream, it will destroy a substance called hemoglobin that the blood uses to transport oxygen throughout the body. This is why it's especially important to focus on relaxed breathing that comes from the diaphragm.

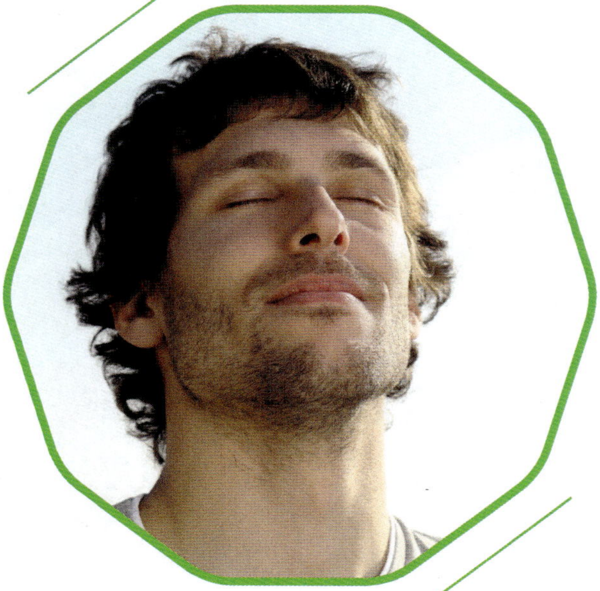

How to Breathe Correctly

The easiest way to relearn correct breathing is to lie flat on your back on the floor, on a mat or blanket or on a firm bed. Place a small weighted object on your belly button, like a heavy book. Take a deep breath in through your nose so that the book rises as your stomach, or diaphragm, fills with air. Hold this deep breath for a count of 4 and then release through your nose so that your stomach deflates. Use this process to release any tension as you exhale and repeat. In the exercise, your chest should not move to indicate relaxed, stress-free breathing.

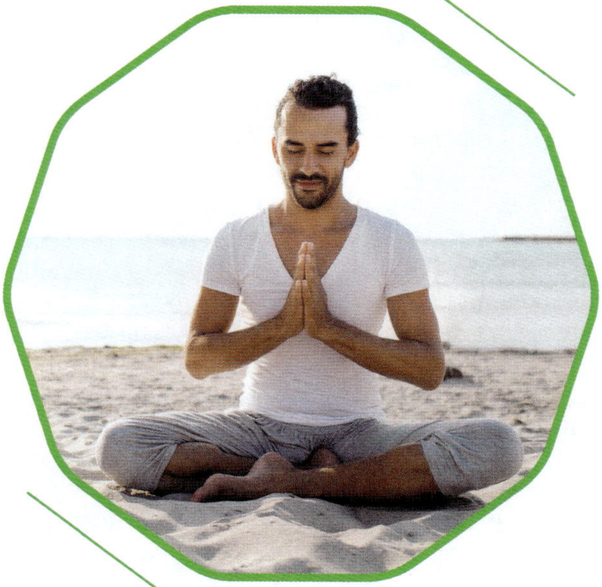

♂ Practice this low-stress breathing exercise again and again as you lie down. Once you have mastered the rhythm of the calming breath, you can start to try the exercise while standing. Initially, you may feel dizzy as you intake more and more fresh oxygen, but it's still important to practice the exercise whenever you can.

9. Stimulate Acupressure Points

Another component in your Rehabilitation Plan is to stimulate acupressure points that connect to your health recovery system. There are a number of points that can be massaged gently with a finger to mimic actual acupuncture. Please read more about this on **page 41**.

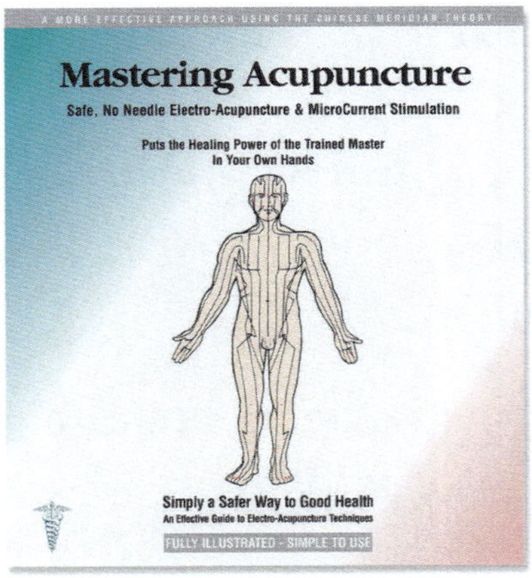

10. Get More Sun Exposure

An essential vitamin to support your overall health is vitamin D3. You can find a large dose of vitamin D3 in the recommended supplement on **page 38**, but it's still critical to get some natural vitamin D from sun exposure.

The sun is the source of life. Unfortunately, myths have been circulated in the health community that the sun is an enemy that we must stay away from at all costs. Even worse, many health professionals recommend slathering your body in toxic chemicals every time you go out in the sun. Of course, I'm not recommending lying in the sun for 6 hours at once on the first hot day of the year. It's essential to build up the skin's tolerance to sun exposure over several weeks for natural protection. By the time that hot summer days come around, you will be able to tolerate a greater amount of natural sun exposure.

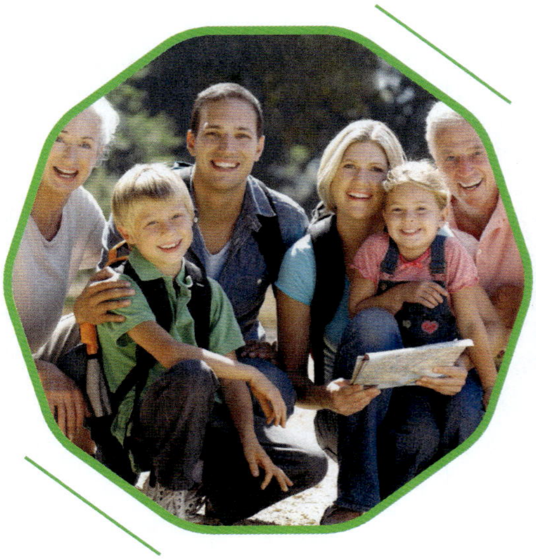

Recommendations:

A. Get as much skin exposed to the sun as you can every day, e.g. on your daily walk.

B. Build up slowly from the spring to summer time.

C. Try not to stay out in the middle of the day without covering up, and cover up rather than use a barrier cream.

D. If you do use a sun cream, get an organic one rather than chemical ones with well-known names.

E. Remember, the sun is your friend, and as with friends, try not to get too much in one go!

More About Clearing Inflammation and Promoting Healing

Prostate Plus+

If you're male and over 40, you *must* consider looking after your prostate health! Start with a powerful non-drug, *natural* vitamin, herb, and mineral formula with activating enzymes for maximum absorption. Prostate Plus+ is a combination of 23 important nutrients designed to help prostate problems and maintain men's health.

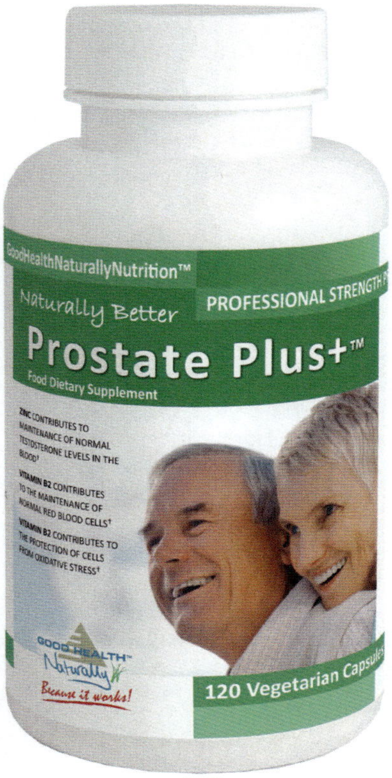

Ingredients:

- Vitamin A (from beta-Carotene) -1230 IU, 25%
- Vitamin E (a-alpha Tocopherols) -100 IU, 333%
- Vitamin B2 - 4 mg, 300%
- Vitamin B6 - 48 mg, 3800%
- Vitamin D3 -1200 IU, 200%
- Copper (from Copper Glycinate Chelate) - 600 mcg,30%
- Zinc (from L-OptiZinc 20%) - 10 mg, 125%
- Selenium (from L-Selenomethinione) -140 mcg, 200%
- Pomegranate Powder Extract - 260mg, 40%
- Saw Palmetto Extract - 200 mg, 45%
- Nettle Root Extract - 180 mg, 2%
- Uva Ursi Extract - 108 mg, 20%
- Graminex G63 -108 mg
- L-Glycine - 90 mg
- L-Alanine - 90 mg
- Lycored Beadlets - 60 mg, 5%
- Panax Ginseng Extract 10:1 -18 mg
- Proprietary Blend -560 mg
- Asparagus Extract 5:1, Blessed Thistle Powder, Damiana Extract 5:1, Fenugreek Seed Powder, Cayenne Powder 40,000HU, Marshmallow Root Powder

Other Ingredients:

Vegetable cellulose (Capsule), Rice Bran and Medium Chain Triglycerides

Dosage:
Take 2 capsules daily

Serranol

The secret behind Serranol is the distinct combination of four key ingredients: Curcumin X4000, Ecklonia Cava Extract, Serrapeptase, and Vitamin D3. In one vegetarian capsule, these core nutrients provide a super-supplement that studies show targets dozens of health and aging-related issues.

- **Serrapeptidase** (technically Serriatia Peptidase) is a diverse proteolytic enzyme that will dissolve non-living tissue, including blood clots, cysts, scarring, plaque, fibrin, and all types of inflammation, without causing harm to living tissue in the body. Serrapeptidase can be used to enhance your overall wellbeing, ease inflammation, and support health to benefit the lungs, joints, digestive tract, colon, arteries, and any other areas of blockage/inflammation.
- **Curcumin** (CurcuminX4000) is praised as one of the best natural, anti-inflammatory herbs. It can stimulate glutathione in the body to guard healthy cells and tissues against inflammation, while moderating the immune system. Curcumin is also known for its antiviral, antifungal, and antibacterial properties.
- **Ecklonia Cava** (Seanol®) has been used by the Asian population for centuries as a type of edible brown algae called Ecklonia Cava Extract. It is harvested off the coast of China, Korea, and Japan; studies support that ECE offers a wide range of health benefits.
- **Vitamin D3** is an essential vitamin to support immune health. Cells in the immune system are made up of vitamin D3 receptors. If there is a deficiency in vitamin D3, it will weaken the immune system and leave the body susceptible to infection. Unfortunately, vitamin D3 deficiency is becoming far too common amongst all age groups since our culture spends far less time in the sun. This valuable vitamin cannot be stored by the body, so daily supplementation is necessary for immune health.

Ingredients:

- **Curcuminx4000 (from Meriva® Curcuma longa extract) - 250mg**
- **Ecklonia Cava Extract 25:1 - 50mg**
- **Serrapeptase - 80,000IU**
- **Vitamin D3 - 1000IU**

Other Ingredients:

Microcrystalline Cellulose, Hypromellose, water, gellan gum (DR capsule)

Dosage:

Take 2 capsules x 3 times per day. Take 30 minutes before eating a meal with water. Reduce to 1 x 3 after a good relief.

Nascent Iodine Drops

Nascent Iodine is totally different from the typical iodine in its denser state sold as an antiseptic, as iodine tri-chloride (claiming to be atomized), or as added to potassium iodide to make it soluble in liquid. Nascent Iodine is a consumable iodine in its atomic form rather than its molecular form. It can provide benefits in thyroid and immune support, detoxification, metabolism, improved energy, and more.

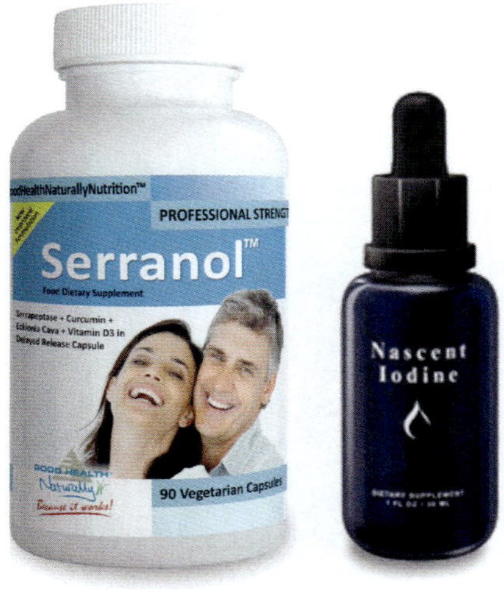

Ingredients:

- **Iodine (in its atomic form) - 400mcg**
- ***2% Iodine by weight***

Other Ingredients:

Nascent Iodine in a base of Demeter certified Biodynamic grape alcohol

Dosage:

Take 5 drops x 3 times per day in 20ml of water; swish around the mouth for 30 seconds before swallowing. Build over 2 weeks to 15 x 3 until well and then slowly reduce back to 5 x 3. Take 1st dose on waking, 2nd mid-morning, and 3rd mid-afternoon.

More About Missing Nutrients

Prescript-Assist

Prescript-Assist (P-A) is a third-generation combination of 29 probiotic microflora Soil-Based-Organisms (SBOs), uniquely joined with a humic/fulvic acid prebiotic that enhances SBO proliferation. Prescript-Assist's microflora are Class-1 micro-ecological units that are typical of those progressively found resident along the healthy human GI tract.

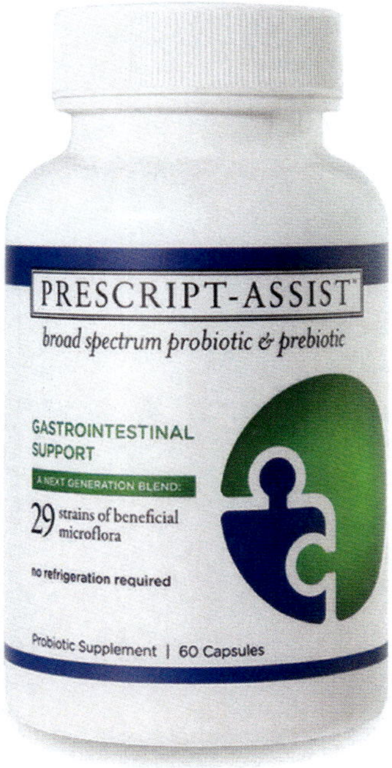

Ingredients:

Contains a proprietary blend of Leonardite and the following Class I (beneficial microorganisms):

- ***Anthrobacter agilis, Anthrobacter citreus, Anthrobacter globiformis, Anthrobacter luteus, Anthrobacter simplex, Acinetobacter calcoaceticus, Azotobacter chroococcum, Azotobacter paspali, Azospirillum brasiliense, Azospirillum lipoferum, Bacillus brevis, Bacillus marcerans, Bacillus pumilis, Bacillus polymyxa, Bacillus subtilis, Bacteroides lipolyticum, Bacteriodes succinogenes, Brevibacterium lipolyticum, Brevibacterium stationis, Kurtha zopfil, Myrothecium verrucaria, Pseudomonas calcis, Pseudomonas dentrificans, Pseudomonas flourescens, Pseudomonas glathei, Phanerochaete chrysosporium, Streptomyces fradiae, Streptomyces celluslosae, Streptomyces griseoflavus***

Other Ingredients:

Cellulose (vegetarian capsule)

Dosage:

Take 1 capsule, 2 times a day.

More About Immune Strengthening Formulations

Active Life

Active Life is an all-natural source of 90 vitamins, minerals, and other nutrients. It comes in a liquid formula to ensure you get all the essential vitamins and minerals needed by your body. This single liquid supplement allows for maximum absorption and utilization in the body - 300% more absorbent than tablets!

Ingredients	Amount per Serving
Calories	39
Calcium (Tricalcium Phosphate, Citrate)	600mg
Choline Bitartrate	25mg
Chromium (Chromium Polynicotinate)	200mcg
Copper (Copper Gluconate)	2mg
Folic Acid (Vitamin B Conjugate)	500mcg
Inositol	50mg
Magnesium (Citrate Gluconate Concentrate)	300mg
Manganese (Manganese Gluconate)	10mg
Organic Seleniumethionine	200mcg
Potassium (Potassium Gluconate)	250mg
Vitamin A (Palmitate)	5000IU
Vitamin A (Beta Carotene)	5000IU
Vitamin B1 (Thiamine Mononitrate)	3mg
Vitamin B12 (Methylcobalamin)	6mcg
Vitamin B2 (Riboflavin)	3.4mg
Vitamin B3 (Niacinamide)	40mg
Vitamin B5 (Calcium Pantothenate)	20mg
Vitamin B6 (Pyridoxine Hydrochloride)	4mg
Vitamin C (Ascorbic Acid)	300mg
Vitamin D (Cholecalciferol)	400IU
Vitamin E (Alpha Tocopheryl Acetate)	60IU
Vitamin K (Phytonadione)	80mcg
Zinc (Oxide)	15mg
Ionic Trace Minerals	600mg
Phosphorus (Amino Acid Chelate)	190mg
Biotin	300mcg
Iodine (Potassium Iodine)	150mcg
Boron (Sodium Borate)	2mg
Molybdenum	75mcg
Chloride Concentrate	102mg
Amino Acid Complex	10mg
Aloe Vera Extract (200:1)	2 mg

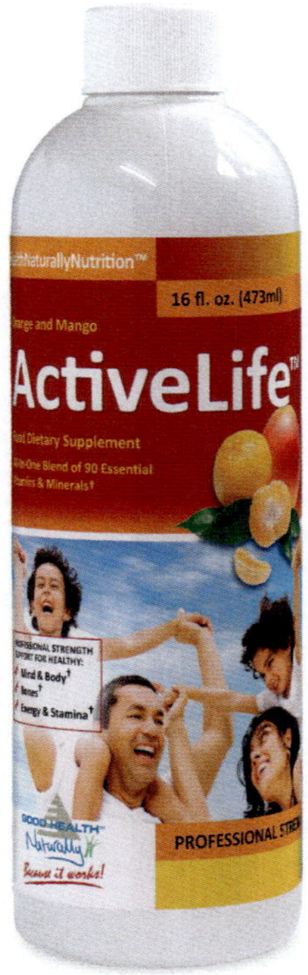

Dosage:

Take 15ml x 2 times daily with meals.

In a liquid base of:

Purified Water, Natural Vegetable Glycerine, Mixed Fruit Concentrate (Peach, Pear, Pineapple), Natural Flavors Blend, Xanthan Gum, Citric Acid, Potassium Sorbate (for freshness).

Allergen Info: Contains Corn. GLUTEN FREE.

More About Optional Nutrients

1st Line Immune Support Kit

1st Line is a new all-natural product designed to fight against many types of infections, including viruses. It is a patented formula by a British chemist containing Thiocyanate Ions. When added to water, 1st Line provides a drink which forms the same molecules that make up our body's first line of defense against all types of bacteria, yeast, fungi, flu, germs, and viruses. 1st Line offers an aggressive attack on these unwanted infections without doing harm to healthy bacteria in the body, a common side effect when using antibiotic drugs. 1st Line is safe and easy to use.

Ingredients:

- **Sodium Thiocyanate - 100ppm**
- **Sodium Hypothiocyanate - 60ppm**

Other Ingredients:

Hydrogen Peroxide, Poly Aluminium Chloride, Lactoperoxidase, and Bentonite. Note that no hydrogen peroxide or aluminum is consumed as these are converted by the enzymes in the creation of the oxythiocyanate ions or are residues in the green/brown mass.

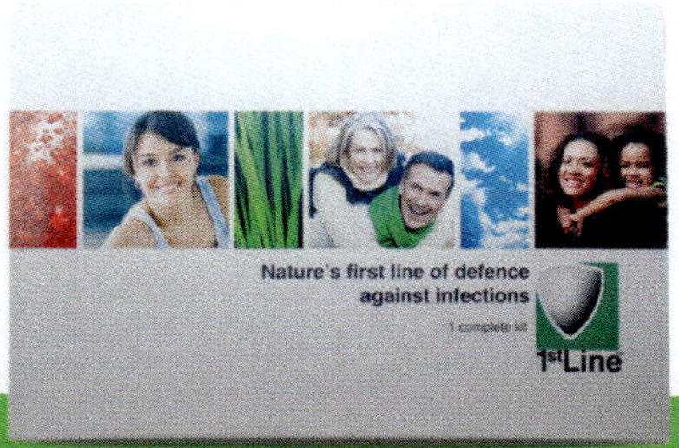

Dosage:

Always take at least 90 minutes before and 90 minutes after food. Take 1 kit daily for 3 days (a total of 3). ***Three kits should be taken as a minimum; in serious conditions, 10 kits are better if finances allow.***

More About Acupressure

Stimulating the points in page 7.2 of the book **Mastering Acupuncture** will help to balance men's health. These points can be effectively and safely stimulated using the **HealthPoint™** electro-acupressure kit. The advantage of the kit is it gives you the power to precisely locate the acupuncture point, and indeed other points, so you can enjoy the benefits of acupuncture at home and without any needles.

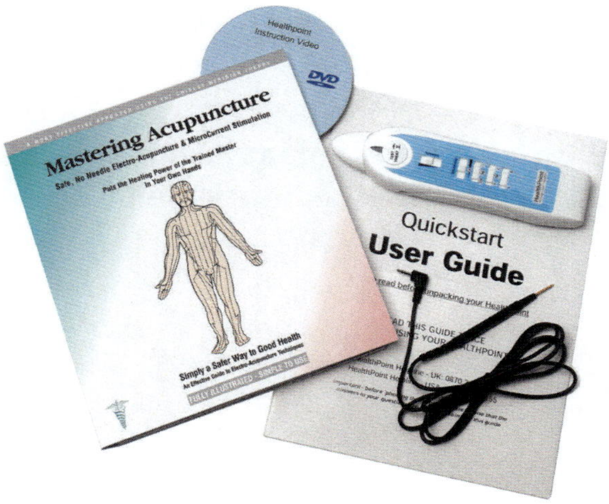

HealthPoint™ is easy to use, painless, and effective. It includes an instructional DVD and book covering over 150 pain and non-pain conditions that can be helped, such as headaches, back, neck, and joint problems.

The gentle and systematic stimulation of the body's natural healing system can speed recovery in many cases. **HealthPoint™** breakthrough technology was developed by leading pain control specialist Dr. Julian Kenyon MD 21 years ago, and today features the latest microchip technology to quickly locate acupuncture points key to specific health conditions, such as the points for men's health recovery.

In Conclusion:

The Men's Health Rehabilitation Program offers a complete rehabilitation plan that is specially designed to comprehensively prevent or manage your men's health condition.

Men's health issues and diseases can better be understood as lifestyle diseases. This means that if you change your lifestyle, there is a great chance of partial or full recovery. When you implement the changes found in the 10 Step Plan, your body can naturally begin the healing process to recover your health.

♂ Drugs don't make you healthy.

Drugs aren't effective since they can't make you healthy again. In a best-case scenario, drugs may provide some relief. In a worst-case scenario, they will further damage your health and can even cause untimely death.

Of course, the pharmaceutical industry would love you to continue on your current drug regimen and ineffective rehabilitation plan, relying on toxic medications that inhibit your true path to long-term healing.

♂ Thankfully, you have discovered that there is a better way.

You can use the Men's Health Rehabilitation Program to prevent or manage men's health conditions, even if other medical alternatives have not worked for you:

- This program will help you to embrace your health and improve your quality of life in a rehabilitation plan that includes education, coaching, and exercise.
- This program will incorporate support and therapy to provide assistance so that you can achieve the best results possible.

You will find the Men's Health Rehabilitation Program outlined in this book. When you follow it carefully, you will see some results starting within weeks.

♂ This rehabilitation plan will always offer health improvements.

The worst outcome when using this plan will be that your health improves, but you still need to take some drugs if your health has been damaged irreparably by medication or illness.

♂ Start slowly and begin rehabilitation step-by-step.

Unless you are already used to making changes in your life, you will find adopting these habits of healthy living can be difficult to sustain. Persist. Because...

♂ Your health is invaluable.

Robert Redfern, Your Health Coach

Email: robert@goodhealth.nu
www.MyGoodHealthClub.com
for step-by-step coaching and support.

Men's Health Daily Rehabilitation Plan

TIME	ACTION	AMOUNT
OPTIONAL ITEMS		
Just before eating	1st Line Kit	Take 1 kit daily for 3 days. It should be taken 90 minutes before and 90 minutes after food, approximately.
BREAKFAST		
30 minutes before breakfast	Serranol	Take 2 capsules, with water
With breakfast	Prostate Plus+	Take 1 capsule
With breakfast	Active Life	Take 15ml with water
With breakfast	Nascent Iodine Drops	Take 5 drops in 20ml of water
LUNCH		
30 minutes before lunch	Serranol	Take 2 capsules, with water
With lunch	Active Life	Take 15ml with water
With lunch	Prescript-Assist	Take 1 capsule
With lunch	Nascent Iodine Drops	Take 5 drops in 20ml of water
EVENING MEAL		
30 minutes before evening	Serranol	Take 2 capsules, with water
With your evening meal	Prostate Plus+	Take 1 capsule
With your evening meal	Prescript-Assist	Take 1 capsule
With your evening meal	Nascent Iodine Drops	Take 5 drops in 20ml of water

Other Recommended Books for Health Recovery:

- Improving Lung Health in 30 Days
- Solving Diabetes Type 2 in 27 Days
- Improving Kidney Health in 30 Days
- Improving Multiple Sclerosis in 30 Days
- Improving Arthritis in 30 Days
- Improving Heart Disease in 30 Days
- Improving Stroke in 30 Days
- Improving Alzheimer's Disease in 30 Days

Other Books by Robert Redfern:

- The 'Miracle Enzyme' Is Serrapeptase
- Turning A Blind Eye
- Mastering Acupuncture
- EquiHealth Equine Acupressure

Made in the USA
Las Vegas, NV
11 November 2025

34061258R10029